ROLE OF CATECHOLAMINES
IN
CARDIOVASCULAR DISEASES

Role of Catecholamines

in

Cardiovascular Diseases

I. HYPERTENSION

Professor of Physiology and Pharmacology
St. Louis University Medical School
St. Louis, Missouri U.S.A.

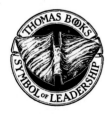

CHARLES C THOMAS · PUBLISHER
Springfield · Illinois · U. S. A.

Published and Distributed Throughout the World by

CHARLES C THOMAS • PUBLISHER

Bannerstone House

301-327 East Lawrence Avenue, Springfield, Illinois, U.S.A.

© *1974, by* CHARLES C THOMAS • PUBLISHER

ISBN 0-398-02900-8

Library of Congress Catalog Card Number: 73-7759

*With THOMAS BOOKS careful attention is given to all details of manu-
facturing and design. It is the Publisher's desire to present books that are
satisfactory as to their physical qualities and artistic possibilities and
appropriate for their particular use. THOMAS BOOKS will be true to
those laws of quality that assure a good name and good will.*

Printed in the United States of America

EE-11

Library of Congress Cataloging in Publication Data
Bhagat, Budh Dev.
  Role of catecholamines in cardiovascular diseases.
  CONTENTS: v. 1. Hypertension.
    1. Cardiovascular system—Diseases. 2. Catecholamines. I. Titles.
[DNLM: 1. Cardiovascular diseases—Drug therapy. 2. Catecholamines—
Therapeutic use. WG166 B575r 1973]
RC669.B46   616.1'3   73-7759
ISBN 0-398-02900-8

Dedicated
to
My Mother, Subdhra Devi Bhagat
with Gratitude and Appreciation for
Her Invaluable Guidance in All of my Endeavors

PREFACE

This book provides an up-to-date link between the biochemistry and pharmacology of antihypertensive drugs and their relation to clinical practice.

The etiology of hypertension is far from complete. Drugs such as reserpine and guanethidine that affect the storage and release of norepinephrine are being used successfully in the treatment of hypertension. This fact, together with the recent observations that plasma catecholamines are elevated in patients with essential hypertension, indicate the involvement of the sympathetic nervous system in the pathogenesis of hypertension. Furthermore, the turnover rate of norepinephrine in the central and peripheral nervous systems are increased in animals with experimentally produced hypertension. This book integrates and clarifies our present knowledge of the role of neurohormones in the causation of hypertension.

This book has been divided into three main sections. The first section deals with catecholamines, the second with their influence on the cardiovascular system and the third with hypertension. The section on the cardiovascular system has been included with the idea that an understanding of the normal physiological processes will make a great impact on the approach to the treatment of hypertension.

In planning, I have used what seemed to me the most practical if not always most logical arrangement. The reader should attribute the distribution of emphasis and space in the text to the interest, experience, capacities and prejudices of the author.

Space limitation in this book restricts the provision of full credit which is due all of the investigators whose papers have contributed to the present understanding of the subject. I have also taken considerable liberties in the reviewing and interpretation of the material covered.

This book is written for general practitioners, interns, residents, medical students, research workers and nurses interested in cardiology, particularly hypertension. Specialists will find this book a useful means of keeping abreast of new adrenergic drugs and knowledge of their mechanism of action. May this book improve the approach to the treatment of hypertension.

I wish to express my appreciation to Drs. A.R. Lind, L.S. D'Agrosa, Sham Gandhi and K. Christensen for their many suggestions and advice relative to the preparation of this monograph. To Pamela J. Dockins I give my special thanks for typing the manuscript under most trying conditions. I also thank my niece, Adell Levine, whose sufferings during open heart surgery motivated me to write on cardiovascular diseases. Finally I am grateful to Mr. Donald E. Biggerstaff for most of the art work presented in this book.

Budh Dev Bhagat

CONTENTS

Page

Dedication v

Preface vii

Chapter

THE CATECHOLAMINES
SECTION ONE

I. Distribution, Location and Function 3
    Development of Transmitter concept 4
    Storage of norepinephrine 7
    Release of norepinephrine 9
    Adrenal Medullary catecholamines 10

II. Fate of Released Catecholamine 12
    Relative importance of catechol-O-methyl transferase
        and monoamine oxidase in metabolism of norepinephrine 13
    Relative importance of binding and metabolism of
        norepinephrine 15
    Steps in uptake of amine 16
    Importance of uptake 20
    Inactivation of norepinephrine in vascular tissue 21
    Extraneuronal uptake 23

III. Biosynthesis of Catecholamines 26
    Rate limiting step in biosynthesis of norepinephrine 28
    Regulation of synthesis of norepinephrine 29

IV. False Neurotransmitters 34
    Synthesis of false neurotransmitter 34
    Physiological consequence of accumulation false
        neurotransmitter 37

V. Summary of events at adrenergic neuroeffector Organs 38

SECTION TWO
THE CARDIOVASCULAR SYSTEM

VI. Heart 45
    Contractility of the heart 49
    Innervation of the heart 53

VII. Blood Vessels 58
    Structure of vessels 58
    Control of calibre of blood vessels 60
    Circulation in the skin 73
    Circulation in the skeletal muscle 74

VIII. Regulation of Blood Pressure 77
    Baroreceptor funcion 77
    Medullary control 77
    Hormonal control of the cardiovascular system 83

Chapter		Page
	Circulatory changes during muscular exercise	91
	Long term control of blood pressure	93
IX.	Renin and Angiotensin System	98
X.	Prostaglandins	104
XI.	Adrenergic Receptors	108
	Classification of adrenergic receptors	109
	Classification of β-receptors	110
	Physiological significance of β-receptors	114
XII.	Actions of Norepinephrine, Epinephrine and Other Amines on the Cardiovascular System	118

SECTION THREE
HYPERTENSION

XIII.	Hypertension and Treatment	127
	Labile hypertension	129
	Sustained hypertension	129
	Neurogenic hypertension	131
	Aldosteronism	135
	Renovascular hypertension	140
	Role of sympathetic nervous system in human hypertension	142
	Effects of hypertension	144
	Program of treatment	146
	Hypertensive emergencies	156
XIV.	Pheochronocytoma	158
	Diagnosis	159
	Treatment	161
XV.	Pharmacology of Antihypertensive Agents	163
	Ganglionic blocking agents	163
	Reserpine	164
	Alpha methyldopa (Aldomet)	169
	Guanethidine	173
	MAO inhibitors (Pargyline)	176
	Thiazide (diuretics)	177
	Hydralazine	181
References		185
Index		197

SECTION ONE

THE

CATECHOLAMINES

CHAPTER I

DISTRIBUTION,

LOCATION AND FUNCTION

THE WORD "CATECHOLAMINES" applies to any compound which has a catechol nucleus (a benzene ring with two adjacent hydroxyl groups) and an amine-containing side chain.

Naturally Occurring Catecholamine

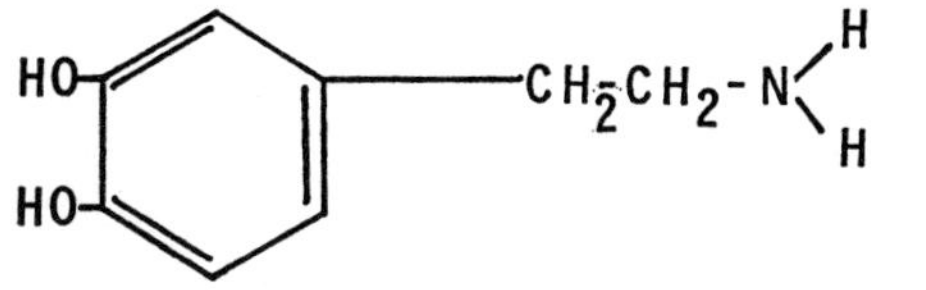

DOPAMINE

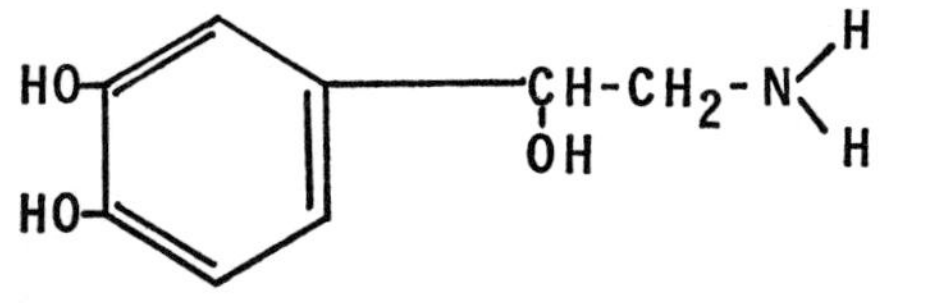

NOREPINEPHRINE

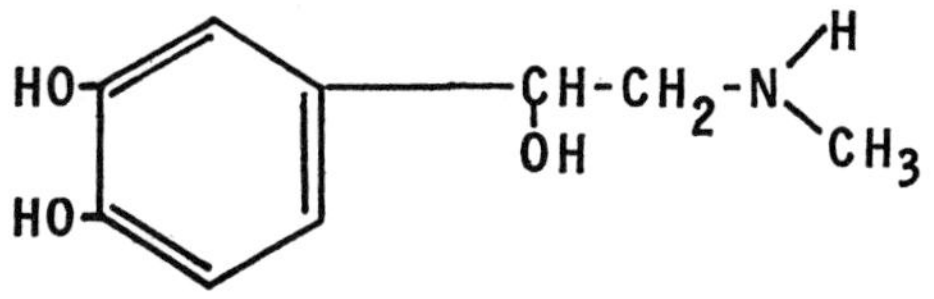

EPINEPHRINE

There are three naturally occurring catecholamines: dopamine, norepinephrine and epinephrine. Dopamine has been demonstrated in the adrenal medulla (Goodall, 1950, 1951) and in various organs (Von Euler and Lishajko, 1957; Angelkos *et al.,* 1963; Bjorklund *et al.,* 1970), including the central nervous system (Montagu, 1957; Bertler and Rosengren; 1959, Sano *et al.,* 1959; Hornykiewicz, 1966). Dopamine serves not only as a precursor for norepinephrine, but also occurs as a chromaffin cell hormone in "dopamine cells" in various organs (Falck *et al.,* 1959), in the adrenal (Eade, 1958; Lishajko, 1969; 1970a) and in the carotid body (Chiocchio *et al.,* 1966; Lishajko, 1970b). In the central nervous system it is present as a neurotransmitter (Fuxe, 1965). Histochemical and biochemical studies have revealed the presence of separate neuronal cells in the central nervous system in which dopamine is predominant rather than norepinephrine. Dopamine-containing neurons are particularly abundant in the striatum (Hornykiewicz, 1966).

Norepinephrine is the neurotransmitter and is present mainly in the sympathetic nerves of the peripheral system and of the central nervous system. If released it acts locally on the effector cells of the smooth muscle of blood vessels, adipose tissue, liver, heart and brain.

Epinephrine is mostly found in the chromaffin cells of the adrenal medulla. It is released as a hormone and acts on many distant effector cells via the blood stream.

Development of Transmitter Concept

There is a similarity between the effect of drugs and those of nerve stimulation. For example, when muscarine is applied to the heart, it slows it in a manner similar to vagal stimulation.

In 1895, Oliver and Schafer showed that the adrenal extract mimicked the effects of sympathetic stimulation. Therefore, they suggested that sympathetic nerves may act by releasing a chemical substance. Although this idea was interesting, it was not universally accepted.

In 1905 Elliot wrote "the reaction to adrenaline of any plain muscle in the body is of a similar character to that following excitation of the sympathetic nerves supplying that muscle" and further, "that when plain muscle develops connections with sympathetic nerves it must, at the myoneural junction, acquire a mechanism that can receive the nervous impulse and thereupon initiate the appropriate muscular response. That part of the junction which is irritated by adrenaline is on the muscular side." However, the convincing evidence that chemical transmission occurs was provided by Loewi in 1921. He perfused two isolated frog hearts with Ringer's solution in such a way that the solution flowed through one heart, perfusing the other. When the vagus nerve of the first heart was stimulated, the heart slowed and shortly afterward the second heart behaved in a similar manner. On the basis of these results he suggested that during stimulation of the vagus, a substance was released from the nerve endings which slowed the first heart. When this substance was carried in the perfusion fluid to the second heart, it arrested the second heart also. He called this substance "vagusstoff." By similar experiments, he was also able to show that stimulation of the nervus accelerans caused the release of an accelerator substance called "acceleranstoff." Subsequent work established the fact that the "vagusstoff" was acetylcholine and "acceleranstoff" was epinephrine or norepinephrine (Von Euler, 1948; Pearts, 1949).

Following these discoveries, it became apparent that drugs which mimic the effects of nerves must be acting on the effector cells directly and not through an action on the nerve endings.

Synapse.

Electron microscopy has revealed that axon terminal (pre-synaptic) does not fuse with the effector cell (post-synaptic). Pre- and post-synaptic cells are separated by a gap usually 200 to 600 Å. Some postganglionic sympathetic axons may be separated from the effector cells they innervate by as much as several microns. The gap between the pre- and post-synaptic cells is termed the synaptic cleft. It is this characteristic which clearly separates chemically transmitting and electrically coupled synapses, since the electrical type commonly shows fusion of pre- and post-synaptic membranes (Pappas and Bennet, 1966). During the process of synaptic chemical transmission, an electrical signal in the pre-synaptic cell causes the release of a transmitter into the synaptic cleft where it interacts with a specific site (called a **receptor**) on the post-synaptic site to cause a mechanical response.

Sympathetic Neuron.

The sympathetic postganglionic neurons arise from cell bodies in the paravertebral and the prevertebral ganglia and extend to the effector organs, where they are distributed in a network of terminations which lack the specificity of the neuroeffector junction seen in the motor end plate of voluntary nerves and skeletal muscle. Recently, it has been possible to examine the anatomic distribution of the sympathetic postganglionic fibers in considerable detail. With the development of sensitive histochemical methods, specific identification of adrenergic neurons has become possible.

It is now believed that, morphologically, an adrenergic neuron may be divided into three different regions: cell body, axon and nerve terminal (Fig. 1A).

THE CELL BODY. This is usually located in the autonomic ganglia of the sympathetic trunks and the pre-vertebral ganglia (celiac, superior mesenteric and inferior mesenteric) but it can also be found in some intra-mural ganglia, for example, in the wall of the urinary bladder (Norberg and Hamberger, 1964). Each cell body (diameter about 30 μ) contains ribosomes, Golgi material and other usual cytoplasmic organelles.

THE AXON. From each cell body one long unmyelinated nerve fiber arises. It is usually 0.2 to 1 μ in diameter and is quite simple in structure, containing primarily neurofilaments, neurotubules and mitochondria. Often 5 to 10 or more fibers run together enclosed within the depressions of the cell membrane of one Schwann cell.

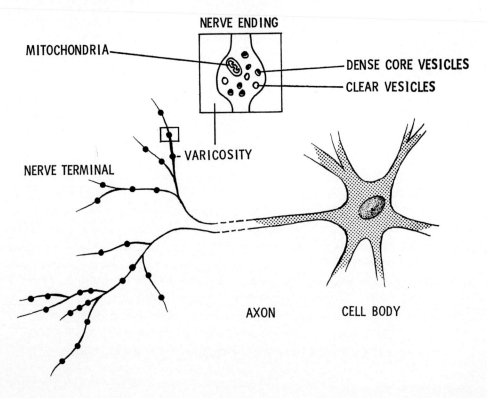

THE NERVE TERMINAL. When the axon approaches the tissue to be innervated, it becomes varicose. In the innervated tissue each axon splits into
a system of branches called nerve terminals. The terminal fibers of one
neuron run in bundles together with the terminal fibers of other neurons.
They form a ground plexus (Hillarp, 1946) which is supported by a network of Schwann cells. Thus, each adrenergic fiber innervates many effector
cells and each effector cell is innervated by many adrenergic fibers which
originate from different neurons. The average total length of the terminal
system of each neuron is about 10 cm (Dahlström and Häggendal, 1966 a,b).
These ramifications of the axons are the true terminals. They often form
basket-like arrangements around the innervated components. On these
terminals, at regular intervals, are bead-like structures called varicosities.
The release of the neurotransmitter, norepinephrine, is believed to occur
from these varicose enlargements, where the neurotransmitter is stored in
high concentration in storage particles.

Varicosities are usually believed to be pre-synaptic structures from which
the norepinephrine is released in response to a nerve stimulus (Ańden *et al.*,
1969). In some tissues there may be frequent and very close association of
the terminal nerve and the muscle cell membrane, but without any direct
modification of the contact area in the membrane. In other tissues, this
association between nerve and muscle may be less intimate, and the neurotransmitter may be released into the general vicinity of several effector cells.

STORAGE OF NOREPINEPHRINE

Norepinephrine in the adrenergic neuron is stored in axon terminals. However, very small amounts are also present in the cell bodies and pre-terminal axons of the post-ganglionic adrenergic neurons. The amine is stored mainly in the vesicles which have a dense core and a diameter of 400 to 600 Å. There are also a few larger granules of about twice that size. In the storage vesicles, norepinephrine is stored in combination with ATP and protein.

The binding of norepinephrine retards its diffusion out of the cell, thereby protecting it from enzymatic destruction by the enzyme, monoamine oxidase (MAO), which is present in the mitochondria.

The storage of norepinephrine in the granules is not specific because these granules can take up and retain other structurally related compounds like octopamine, α-methyl norepinephrine and metaraminol. The uptake process appears to require ATP and Mg^{++}, is temperature dependent and is blocked by reserpine.

The vesicles are not only the site of storage of norepinephrine, but they are also the site of synthesis and release of norepinephrine. They take up dopamine from the cytoplasm (protecting it from oxidation by MAO) where it is β-hydroxylated to norepinephrine by dopamine β-oxidase. The stored norepinephrine is released in response to appropriate physiological stimuli. The newly synthesized norepinephrine remains in an unbound form for a short period and may be preferentially released. Norepinephrine leaving the granules and entering the cytoplasm is mainly oxidatively deaminated by the MAO of the mitochondria. After inhibition of MAO, the released norepinephrine is taken up and stored again, resulting in the elevation of tissue levels of catecholamine. Thus, intraneuronal MAO plays an important role in the regulation of endogenous amine levels. The cytoplasmic level of norepinephrine must be set by the balance between its leakage from the vesicles, its uptake and its destruction by monoamine oxidase (Kopin, 1964).

Mechanisms Involved in Transmitter Storage

In the synaptic vesicles, or any other types of secretory vesicles (Hillarp, 1959; Dean and Hope, 1968), neuro-transmitters and other secretory products are present in very high concentrations (Potter and Axelrod, 1963a, b; Whittaker, 1966). In the adrenal medullary storage vesicles, the amount of intravesicular catecholamine concentration is approximately 0.8M and adrenergic synaptic vesicles, the transmitters, are present at an osmolarity considerably higher than that of the surrounding cytoplasm. Under these conditions, one might expect the vesicles to be unstable in isotonic solution. But this is not the case, since in isotonic solution at 0°C, the isolated medullary granules retain their catecholamines for a few days. This suggests that the stored amines are present in the storage vesicles in some aggregated molecular form that reduces their effective osmolarity. The presence of stoichiometric amounts (1:4) of negatively charged adenosine triphosphate (ATP) in vesicles suggests binary or ternary complex formation with catecholamines (Hillarp, 1959; Stjärne *et al.*, 1970). *In vitro*, such complexes can form between catecholamines and ATP if both are present in high concentration in aqueous solution in the presence of small amounts of bivalent cations such as Ca^{++} or Mg^{++} (Berneis *et al.*, 1969 a, b). However, the precise nature of the complexes formed, either *in vitro* or in intact storage vesicles, remains obscure. Formation of the Norepinephrine-ATP aggregate is inhibited by tyramine or amphetamine, and is also altered by small quantities of reserpine which appears to combine with, and precipitate, some of the system constituents (Berneis *et al.*, 1970). Soluble vesicular proteins, such as chromogranin A, may have some role in a complex formation in adrenergic and adrenal medullary vesicles. Slotkin and Kirshner (1971) believe that chromogranins play a secondary role in the binding of the amines to ATP in the storage complex, perhaps by stabilizing the complex and contributing to the structural specificity of the binding of the various amines in the complex. Other investigations suggest that the sulfhydryl groups of the storage vesicle membrane may play an important role in catecholamine storage (Taugner and Hasselbach, 1968; Keswani, *et al.*, 1969).

Whatever the nature of the storage complex is, it appears to be a loose one, since stored amine in the vesicles can be exchanged with exogenous norepinephrine. There is evidence that a net uptake of exogenous amine or ATP can occur *in vitro* (Smith, 1968; Kirshner, 1969). The ATP present in the granules also serves the purpose of supplying energy for the release of catecholamines (Kirshner, 1969).

AXOPLASMIC TRANSPORT

The large axon of the sympathetic neuron which connects the cell body to distally located and specialized nerve endings, not only conducts nerve impulses but also provides a system for the continual flow of substances from the cell body to the nerve endings. There is immunohistochemical evidence which suggests that the enzymes necessary for the conversion of tyrosine to norepinephrine and the protein components of the vesicles, are synthesized in the cell body and then transported down the axon to the terminals by axoplasmic flow.

When the sympathetic nerve is ligated, endogenous norepinephrine with its granular vesicles, and enzymes, such as dopamine β-oxidase, accumulate above the constriction, but not below the ligation. When two ligations are placed on the same nerve, no accumulation occurs above the second, more distal, constriction. The transport is not bidirectional and seems to be independent of both perikaryon and nerve terminal, since Dahlström, in 1967, found that in an isolated part of the nerve, the transport of granules occurred. The axonal transport is a highly specialized process and various constituents are transported down the axon to the nerve terminal at varying rates. Granules are transported at a rate of 5 to 6 mm per hour and their average life span is 35 to 70 days. This exceeds the time required for the turnover of norepinephrine in the nerve terminal. This suggests that most of the norepinephrine in the terminals is synthesized locally and that granules are reused many times during their life span.

Microtubules have been implicated in the mechanism for rapid axonal transport. It has been shown that mitotic inhibitors, colchicine and vinblastine, which causes disruption of the microtubules, block the somatofugal transport of norepinephrine and dense core vesicles in the sympathetic neurons.

RELEASE OF NOREPINEPRINE

RESTING SECRETION. There is strong evidence that the effector organ is normally under the influence of a *resting secretion* of norepinephrine from the postganglionic sympathetic nerves comparable to the resting secretion of the adrenal medulla. This resting secretion may be visualized as consisting of two components: a) spontaneous random discharge of packets or quanta of norepinephrine, which set up the so-called miniature junction potentials in the effector cells (Burnstock and Holman, 1962) (this phenomenon is clearly visible to the electrophysiologists, but the amount of norepinephrine released is far too small to cause a mechanical response of the effector organ) ; and b) release of relatively large amounts of norepinephrine, as a result of impulse traffic from the central nervous system, which maintain tonic activity, particularly in the vascular smooth muscle.

When the preganglionic fibers of the sympathetic nerve are cut, the spontaneous release of norepinephrine is reduced (Hertting *et al.*, 1962 b) . The spontaneous release of norepinephrine is also diminished by drugs such as ganglionic blocking agents (Hertting *et al;* 1962a; Bhagat, 1963a) adrenergic neuron blocking agents (Bhagat, 1963a) and monamine oxidase inhibitors (Axelrod *et al;* 1961) . The common denominator in all of these experiments appears to be inhibition of the tonic impulses in the sympathetic nerves.

Tonic impulse traffic plays an important role in the depleting action of reserpine (Hertting *et al;* 1962a; Weiner *et al;* 1962; Bhagat, 1963a) . When the synthesis of norepinephrine is inhibited, the physiologic nerve impulse flow causes depletion of tissue norepinephrine stores (Bhagat, 1967) . Since no new norepinephrine is formed, continuous tonic release is sufficient to lead to a gradual depletion of norepinephrine.

RELEASE OF NOREPINEPHRINE BY NERVE IMPULSE. Arrival of a conducted nerve impulse leads to discharge of many quanta and thus causes a mechanical response to the effector organ (Burnstock and Holman, 1962) . It has been estimated that 500 to 1000 molecules of transmitter are released per impulse at a single synapse (Folkow and Häggendal, 1967) . Nerve stimulation appears to release norepinephrine more directly and rapidly into the extraneuronal spaces. De Robertis and Ferreira (1957) have suggested that during nerve stimulation, norepinephrine is released from vesicles located immediately adjacent to the cell membrane at the neuron (Fig. 17). ATP may be lost together with the stored amine. Weiner *et al.*, (1962) showed such a possibility in their experiments on the adrenal medulla.

Farnebo and Hamberger (1970) have recently shown that catecholamine, which accumulates in the cytoplasm following blockade of the Mg^{++}-ATP-dependent-granular storage mechanism by reserpine, is not released by nerve stimulation. These results suggest that transmitter has to be incorporated into the storage granules before it can be released by nerve impulses.

ROLE OF CALCIUM. When an impulse travelling down the nerve fiber invades the nerve terminals, a sequence of events is initiated which terminates in the release of a transmitter. Calcium ions are required for this event. It is usually believed that an impulse makes the membrane of the sympathetic fiber permeable to calcium ions from the extracellular fluid (Fig. 2). The amount of catecholamine released is proportional to the external calcium concentration (Douglas and Rubin, 1963). Kuriyama (1964) found that the size of functional potential induced in smooth muscle by nerve stimulation was increased with an increase in the calcium ion concentration of the bathing medium. Magnesium, which is predominantly an intracellular cation, has an action opposite to that of calcium. When present in an extracellular medium, magnesium competes with calcium for the active sites and depresses the release of norepinephrine in response to sympathetic nerve stimulation. An increase in the calcium concentration partly overcomes the effect of added Mg^{++} (Farmer and Campbell, 1967). The exact role of ions in the release of norepinephrine is poorly understood.

EXOCYTOSIS. Evidence from different laboratories strongly indicates that mechanism of release of catecholamine involves a process of exocytosis, whereby the entire soluble content of the vesicles is discharged to the exterior of the cell. The release of catecholamines is thus accompanied by the release of all other soluble components of granules: adenine nucleotide (ATP) chromagranins and the soluble portions of dopamine β-hydroxylase. However, the release does not involve the extrusion of the entire vesicle as vesicular membranes are not discharged but remain in the cell as discrete structures. Since both small and large molecules are released, it seems that discharge occurs through the cell membrane rather than by diffusion through the cell cytoplasm.

ADRENAL MEDULLARY CATECHOLAMINES

The chromaffin cells of the adrenal medulla are derived embryologically from the neural crest as are the sympathetic neurons. They are viewed as part of the sympathetic adrenergic system, since they secrete epinephrine and norepinephrine into the circulation in response to their preganglionic stimulation. The released catecholamines are carried in the blood to various organs. Thus adrenal medullary catecholamines subserve a purely hormonal function.

The relative proportion of norepinephrine-producing and epinephrine-producing cells in chromaffin tissue varies rather markedly with the species and with age. In the adult human, roughly 80 percent of the total catecholamine content of the adrenal medulla is epinephrine.

The adrenal medullary catecholamine is retained in larger (200 to 300 mμ) particles, whereas the adrenergic neuron contains small catecholamine storage particles (30 to 60 mμ).

Experimental studies have indicated that differential release of norepinephrine and epinephrine may be produced to different stress stimuli. For example, hypoglycemia can effect specific release of epinephrine whereas decreased blood pressure causes release of both amines. Rubin and Miele (1968) showed that in the cat's perfused adrenal gland catecholamine composition in the perfusate was a function of the duration of the stimulation. It is likely that minimal stimulation of the adrenal medulla releases epinephrine and with more intense stimulation, epinephrine and norepinephrine are both released.

Norepinephrine exerts excitatory effect everywhere by acting on adrenoceptors, whereas epinephrine exerts excitatory as well as inhibitory responses. For example, in the vascular bed of the skeletal muscle it acts on receptors mediating vasodilation. In addition epinephrine causes metabolic effects. The most important of these are increased oxygen consumption and elevation of blood sugar, free fatty acid and plasma potassium. The effects of norepinephrine and epinephrine on cardiovascular systems are presented in Fig. (55, 56).

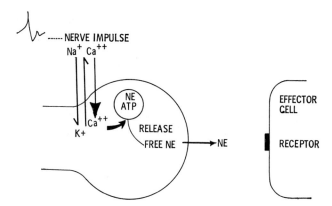

Figure 2. Schematic representation of the events leading to the release of norepinephrine. The arrival of the nerve impulse in the adrenergic nerve terminals causes a series of changes of the ionic permeability of the cell membrane and permits the entry of calcium ions from the extracellular fluid. This entry of calcium ions causes, in some unknown way, the release of norepinephrine.

CHAPTER II

FATE OF RELEASED CATECHOLAMINE

THERE IS NO enzyme similar to acetylcholinesterase which can rapidly destroy catecholamines released by sympathetic nerve stimulation. Furthermore, the inactivation of catecholamines involves a number of processes and is not solely dependent on enzymatic degradation. The enzymes

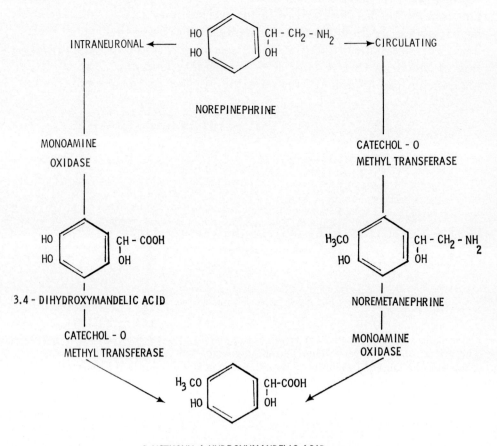

Figure 3. The metabolic pathway of norepinephrine.

principally involved in the inactivation of norepinephrine or epinephrine are monoamine oxidase (MAO) and catechol-O-methyl transferase (COMT).

The catecholamines are almost entirely metabolized in the body, and only small quantities of unchanged amines are found in the urine. Metabolic degradation of catecholamines occurs by way of oxidative deamination and by O-methylation of the catechol nucleus. Mitochondrial monoamine oxidase is responsible for deamination, a pathway which is the predominant one in the neuron, but which also occurs extraneuronally. Catechol-O-methyl-transferase, a soluble cytoplasmic enzyme, appears to be the dominant mechanism of degradation outside the neuron. Both the deaminated and O-methylated metabolites of the catecholamines are substrates for subsequent degradation by the alternate enzymes, and the final common metabolite is 3-methoxy-4-hydroxymandelic acid (vanillylmandelic acid). This metabolic pathway is presented in Figure 3.

Although O-methylated metabolites, metanephrine and normetanephrine represent a smaller fraction of the urinary metabolites of epinephrine and norepinephrine, they are a better measure of the quantity of amines released in a physiologically active form than are the deaminated products. The biotransformation products of dopamine found in the urine are homovanillic acid, a major metabolite, and methoxytyramine. The relative daily excretion of free catecholamines and of their metabolites is roughly: norepinephrine and epinephrine, 0.1 mg; normetanephrine and metanephrine, 1.3 mg; and vanillylmandelic acid, 6.0 mg.

RELATIVE IMPORTANCE OF CATECHOL-O-METHYL TRANSFERASE AND MONOAMINE OXIDASE IN METABOLISM OF NOREPINEPHRINE

The role of MAO and catechol-o-methyl transferase in the metabolism and the inactivation of catecholamines is complex and depends on whether the catecholamine is circulating or bound, as well as on the type of species and tissues involved.

Circulating Catecholamine

In order to study quantitatively the sequential steps in the metabolism of the catecholamines, Axelrod and Tomchick (1958) injected norepinephrine and its metabolite, normetanephrine, into rats and determined the metabolites in the urine. About the same amounts of normetanephrine (free and conjugated) and 3-methoxy-4-hydroxymandelic acid were excreted when either normetanephrine or norepinephrine were administered. When rats were pretreated with a monoamine inhibitor the excretion of 3-methoxy-4-hydroxymandelic acid was reduced and more free and conjugated normetanephrine and norepinephrine were present in the urine. From these observations they concluded that the O-methylation is a major metabolic pathway in the initial metabolism of circulating norepinephrine. The normetanephrine thus formed is subsequently deaminated by monoamine oxidase to yield the major urinary excretion product, 3-methoxy-4-hydroxy-mandelic acid.

Bound Norepinephrine

Bound norepinephrine is released either intraneuronally or into the synaptic cleft; in each case it is metabolized differently. (a) Drugs like reserpine and guanethidine deplete norepinephrine from its storage sites without producing any sympathomimetic response and (b) the norepinephrine is released intracellularly and is deaminated before it leaves the neuron (Kopin and Gordon, 1962, 1963). Thus, there is increased excretion of deaminated catechols.

Drugs like tyramine and other phenylethylamine derivatives deplete norepinephrine stores and cause sympathomimetic activity. In this case, most of the norepinephrine is released into the synaptic cleft. Similarly, drugs which cause stimulation of sympathetic nerves, such as dimethyl-phenylpiperazim (DMPP), nicotine and acetylcholine, release norepinephrine into the circulation. This released norepinephrine, like the injected norepinephrine, is mainly o-methylated.

Uptake of Norepinephrine

Neither of these enzymes is of critical importance in the inactivation of norepinephrine. Inhibition of MAO has no effect on the action of norepinephrine, while inhibition of COMT potentiates it. The physiological activity of catecholamines is mainly terminated by physical mechanisms such as uptake by the axonal membrane and binding within the sympathetic neuron (Hertting, *et al.*, 1961a; Axelrod *et al.*, 1962; Bhagat, 1963b).

When cats were given a tracer dose of ³H-norepinephrine intravenously, killed two minutes later and their tissues examined for labeled norepinephrine, it was found that the labeled catecholamine accumulated in various tissues. The concentration of ³H-norepinephrine was different in various tissues. The highest concentrations were found in organs like the heart and spleen, with rich sympathetic innervation. When the animals were killed two hours after the injection, the concentration of the catecholamine had declined in most tissues, whereas the amount of catecholamines in organs with considerable sympathetic innervation remained high. These results suggest that circulating catecholamines are taken up by the tissue and are retained long after physiological effects of the amine have been dissipated.

The Site of Binding of Catecholamine

When sympathetic nerves are destroyed by chronic denervation, the disappearance of ³H-norepinephrine is very rapid in the denervated organ. Only 10 percent of the initial accumulation remained in the denervated organ 2 hours after injection of ³H-norepinephrine, while 70 percent remained in innervated tissue. These results suggest that the site of uptake of circulating norepinephrine is the sympathetic nerves (Hertting, *et al;* 1961b; Fischer *et al.,* 1965) .

Stjärne *et al.,* (1970) have further shown that this uptake occurs mainly in the nerve terminals, and the uptake in preterminal sympathetic fibers is very low.

THE RELATIVE IMPORTANCE OF BINDING AND METABOLISM OF NOREPINEPHRINE

Thus in the sympathetically innervated organs, catecholamines are inactivated by three mechanisms; (a) uptake and storage in nerve terminal, (b) o-methylation by catechol-o-methyl transferase and (c) oxidative deamination by monoamine oxidase.

The estimates of the partitioning of infused norepinephrine between the various mechanisms of inactivation in perfused cat spleen as shown in Table I, indicates that the majority of norepinephrine is taken up by the adrenergic neuron.

FATE OF INFUSED NOREPINEPHRINE

Uptake by the nerves	60%
Metabolized by O-methyltransferase	15%
Interaction with receptors	5%
Overflow into the circulation (metabolized in liver)	20%

Likewise, histochemical electron-microscopical evidence indicates that inactivation by uptake of norepinephrine is more important than inactivation by metabolism. In support of this is the observation that physiological effects of injected norepinephrine are rapidly terminated, even after both monoamine oxidase and catechol-o-methyl transferase are inhibited (Crout, 1961) .

The Difference Between Dispositions of Norepinephrine and Epinephrine

Whitby *et al.* (1961) found that there are quantitative differences between the disposition of norepinephrine and epinephrine with respect to the rate of uptake, binding and o-methylation. They found that; (a) more ^{3}H-norepinephrine is accumulated than ^{3}H-epinephrine and (b) more o-methylated metabolites are found after epinephrine than after norepinephrine. On the basis of these observations, these investigators have suggested that binding is quantitatively more important for inactivation of norepinephrine, while enzymatic-o-methylation is more important for epinephrine.

This explains why there are higher levels of norepinephrine in the blood than those of epinephrine. The difference is due to their rate of binding rather than to the rate of release into the circulation. Epinephrine is more rapidly metabolized. Similarly, the difference in the rate of uptake may explain why the developed supersensitivity after denervation or after cocaine is greater to norepinephrine than to epinephrine (Trendelenburg, 1965; Bhagat *et al;* 1967).

Steps in the Uptake of Amine

Lindmar and Muscholl (1964) found differences in the rate of uptake and storage of norepinephrine after reserpine. They perfused the rat heart with 20 ng/ml of 1-norepinephrine and determined the rate at which it disappears. They found that the heart removes about 40 percent of the amine, and 98 percent of the removed norepinephrine is then recoverable from the heart.

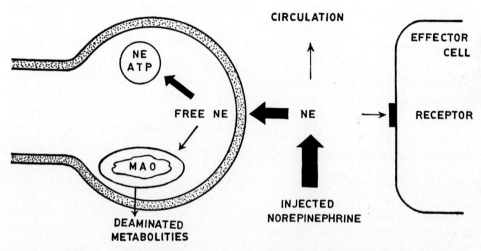

Figure 4. Schematic representation of the fate of 1-norepinephrine at the adrenergic nerve terminal.

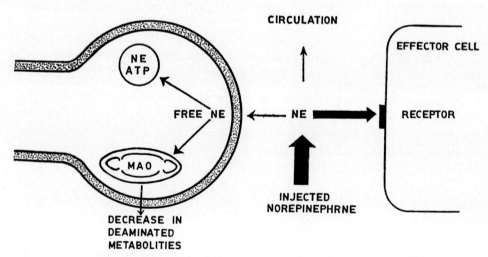

Figure 5. Schematic representation of the effect of pretreatment with cocaine on the effect of 1-norepinephrine at the adrenergic nerve terminal. After administration of cocaine, transport of norepinephrine into the nerve terminal is impaired so that more of the injected norepinephrine is available to act on the adrenergic receptors.

After pretreatment of the rats with reserpine, the removal of norepinephrine remains unaltered, but storage of the removed catecholamine is inhibited.

On the basis of these observations, these investigators concluded that uptake of catecholamines into adrenergic nerve endings is a complex process and involves at least two steps. These are: (a) transport into the nerve terminals and (b) subsequent binding into the norepinephrine stores (Fig.

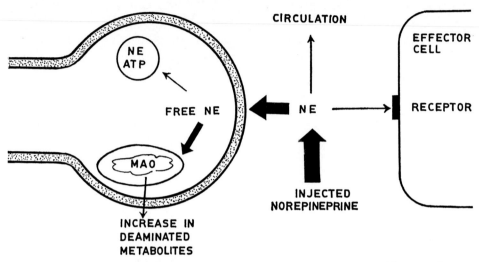

Figure 6. Schematic representation of the effect of pretreatment with reserpine or guanethidine on the fate of l-norepinephrine at the adrenergic nerve terminal. After pretreatment with reserpine or guanethidine, norepinephrine is transported into the nerve terminal at the same rate; but, instead of being stored in intraneuronal vesicles, it is exposed to the action of monoamine oxidase.

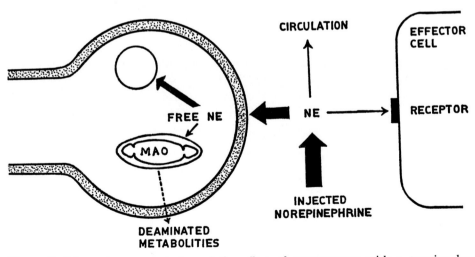

Figure 7. Schematic representation of the effect of pretreatment with a tyrosine hydroxylase inhibitor on the fate of l-norepinephrine at the adrenergic nerve terminal. Storage granules are almost empty, but transport and accumulation of exogenous norepinephrine is normal.

4). Cocaine blocks the uptake of norepinephrine across the neuronal membrane (Fig. 5). The concentration at the receptors remains high and supersensitivity ensues. Reserpine does not interfere with the initial uptake of norepinephrine across the neuronal membrane of sympathetic nerves (Fig. 6). However, the norepinephrine which enters the sympathetic neurons cannot be retained in the normal granule storage site and is rapidly metabolized by monoamine oxidase. This explains why there is no supersensitivity to norepinephrine after treatment with reserpine (short-term).

After pretreatment with a tyrosine hydroxylase inhibitor (Fig. 7), endogenous catecholamines are markedly reduced (Malmfors, 1967; Jonsson, 1969) and storage granules are almost empty (Jonsson and Sachs, 1970). In this case, both uptake and storage of norepinephrine is normal.

The Properties of Norepinephrine Transport

Iversen (1963) has shown that the uptake across the neuronal cell membrane of labeled norepinephrine and epinephrine by the perfused rat heart follows saturation kinetics of the Michaelis-Menten type. Green and Miller (1966) showed that uptake of these amines by strips of rat uterus obeys similar kinetics. The axonal transport mechanism requires energy and is inhibited by ouabain. This process is dependent upon temperature, Na^+ and K^+ (Dengler *et al*; 1962; Bogdanski and Brodie, 1966; Giachetti and Shore, 1966; Iversen and Kravitz, 1966; Gillis and Paton, 1967; Colburn *et al*; 1968; Paton, 1968; Wakade and Furchgott, 1968). It appears that the Na^+- and K^+-activated adenosine triphosphate (membrane ATPase) is involved in the transport of norepinephrine.

All these properties (listed above) are characteristic of active transport of amino acids or sugars across the intestinal epithelium (Crane, 1965; Kipnis and Parrish, 1965). Bogdanski and Brodie (1966), therefore, postulated that the mechanism of uptake of norepinephrine is similar to the Na^+-dependent uptake of sugars and amino acids in other tissues. According to this concept, norepinephrine transport results from an interaction with a membrane carrier whose affinity for the amine is Na^+-dependent. The carrier transports both Na^+ and amine intracellularly where the carrier's affinity for amine is lowered by the low (Na^+) and the high (K^+), thus releasing norepinephrine from the carrier into the cytoplasm of the neuron. The amine is then stored in intraneuronal granules. The inward transport of amine continues since the inward Na^+ gradient is maintained by the extrusion of Na^+ from the cell by means of the pump which is linked to Na^+-K^+-stimulated ATPase (Bogdanski and Brodie, 1969). The transport of amine can be blocked by high (K^+), which antagonizes the high affinity of the carrier in the presence of Na^+, thus blocking inward transport. K^+-free medium prevents the uptake of norepinephrine by inhibiting the ATPase system which in turn results in an increase in intracellular Na^+. The role of ATPase appears to be the maintenance of the ionic gradient.

Amine-uptake—Concentrating mechanisms of the adrenergic neurons.

	OPERATES AT A LEVEL OF NEURONAL MEMBRANE	OPERATES INTRACELLULARLY AT A LEVEL OF AMINE STORAGE GRANULES
INHIBITORS	*COMPETITIVE* COCAINE IMIPRAMINE AND ITS COGENERS GUANETHIDINE BRETYLIUM *NON-COMPETITIVE* OUABAIN	 RESERPINE TETRABENZAINE GUANETHIDINE (LOW DOSES)
SPECIFICITY FOR SUBSTRATE	NON-SPECIFIC	SPECIFIC FOR E-ISOMER OF AMINE
ENERGY REQUIREMENT	Na+-K+ DEPENDENT ATPase	Mg^{2+} DEPENDENT ATPase

Although the reduction of norepinephrine uptake by the adrenergic terminals in the absence of Na+ is considered to be an impairment in the carrier mechanism involved in this process (Bogdanski and Brodie, 1969), other ions such as Ca++ have been shown to influence the action of Na+ in this regard.

Ouabain inhibits amine uptake (Dengler *et al;* 1961; Giachetti and Shore, 1966) in a noncompetitive fashion (Berti and Shore, 1967) since the action of the drug is to decrease the net movement of Na+ across the cell membrane (Glynn, 1964). Cocaine and the tricyclic antidepressants such as imipramine also block uptake, but do so by directly competing with the amine for its attachment site on the carrier (Berti and Shore, 1967). Reserpine does not significantly affect amine transport at the neuron membrane under normal conditions.

Recently, studies by Sugrue and Shore (1970) have revealed the presence of a second Na^+-dependent amine carrier which is separate and distinct from the main reserpine-insensitive and relatively nonspecific amine transport system. This system is optically specific and reserpine-sensitive. The effect of reserpine on this system is short lived. Although the second transport system is located at the axonal membrane and is sodium dependent but requires low sodium similar to those Na^+ concentrations existing intraneuronally.

Granular Uptake

The second step in the uptake process, i.e. the intracellular concentrating mechanism, is presumably located at the granular level and requires Mg^{+2}-dependent ATPase activity. The second transport mechanism is much more specific in its substrate requirement. For example, l-metaraminol and d-metaraminol are substrates for the neuronal membrane amine pump, but only the l-isomer is stored in the granules (Shore *et al;* 1964) . Reserpine, tetrabenazine and low doses of guanethidine inhibit the granular uptake mechanism (Giachetti and Shore, 1969) , while cocaine or imipramine have no effect on this intracellular concentrating mechanism. A comparison of Amine-Uptakes is summarized in Table II.

Importance of Uptake

The importance of initial uptake, i.e. influx of the amine across the neuronal cell membrane, is most important for the termination of the actions. Mg^{+2} ATP-stimulated incorporation is physiologically important for maintaining the catecholamine content of the storage vesicles and for taking up dopamine from the cytoplasm for synthesis of norepinephrine.

The uptake of norepinephrine into nerve terminals removes the amine from the vicinity of the receptors. Normally, rapid uptake keeps the concentrations of injected norepinephrine at the receptors low. When uptake of this amine is impaired, the concentrations at the receptors on the effector organ increase, resulting in an increase in sensitivity (Trendelenburg, 1966) .

When the post-ganglionic sympathetic fibers are cut and time is allowed for the sympathetic fibers to degenerate, the tissue loses its ability to take up and retain norepinephrine. This lack of uptake leads to supersensitivity. Likewise, cocaine impairs the uptake of norepinephrine and causes a similar supersensitivity. In both cases, supersensitivity is the result of availability of more amine at the receptors and not of a change in the response of the effector cell to a given concentration of amine at the receptor (Trendelenburg, 1965) .

Trendelenburg (1966) has further shown that the magnitude of cocaine-induced supersensitivity is proportional to the rate of uptake of the amine. In other words, cocaine should sensitize an effector organ much more to an amine that is taken up rapidly than to an amine that is taken up slowly.

In the isolated atria of the heart (Bhagat *et al;* 1967) and in the nictitating membrane of the spinal cat (Trendelenburg, 1966), cocaine potentiated the action of amines whose magnitude is proportional to the rate of uptake. Cocaine potentiated the responses of an organ to l-norepinephrine more than to l-epinephrine; similarly the relative rates of uptake are: l-norepinephrine less than l-epinephrine (Iversen, 1963). Furthermore, isoproterenol which is hardly taken up at all is not potentiated by cocaine.

Inactivation of Norepinephrine in Vascular Tissue

In the heart and most other sympathetically innervated organs, adrenergic nerve terminals are distributed throughout the entire tissue, whereas the adrenergic innervation of aorta artcries, arterioles, and larger veins is restricted to the adventitia and the underlying portions of the media (Falck, 1962; Pease, 1962; Norberg and Hamberger, 1964). For this reason, in blood vessel the catecholamines are inactivated differently (Fig. 8). Impairment of uptake by either denervation or cocaine causes a relatively smaller degree of super-sensitivity to norepinephrine than that observed for the heart or the nictitating membrane (Bevan and Verity, 1967; Maxwell *et al;* 1968; Trendelenburg *et al;* 1969).

De La Lande and Waterson (1967) determined the site of action of cocaine on the artery. By perfusing the ear artery of the rabbit, they administered norepinephrine either intraluminally or extraluminally and found that cocaine selectively enhanced responses to extraluminal and not to intraluminal norepinephrine. Intraluminally, norepinephrine reaches the smooth muscle of the media before it diffuses to the adrenergic nerve terminals which are confined to the adventitia and the underlying border of the media (adventitio-medial junction). Consequently, intraneuronal uptake is relatively unimportant for the concentration of norepinephrine at the receptor site since sensitivity to norepinephrine is high. Cocaine, therefore, causes only a small degree of supersensitivity. When norepinephrine is administered extraluminally, it reaches the receptors at the edge of the smooth muscular media after having passed the site of uptake (i.e. the nerve endings). As a consequence, the uptake exerts a greater influence on the concentration of the amine at the receptor site, and the sensitivity of the tissue to the amine is low; therefore, cocaine causes marked supersensitivity. Thus they concluded that the action of cocaine on the perfused artery is largely confined to nerves of the adventitia.

Maxwell, *et al;* (1968) showed: 1) approximately 75 percent of the endogenous norepinephrine content of the aorta is in the adventitia; 2) approximately 81 to 90 percent of the capacity of aortic strips to bind norepinephrine resides in the adventitia with the binding sites sensitive to inhibition by cocaine, and 3) the remaining 10 to 20 percent of the capacity for the binding of norepinephrine resides in the media-intimal which is insensitive to inhibition by cocaine. Levin and Furchgott (1970) have suggested that in the adventitia and underlying border of the media, as in any other organ,

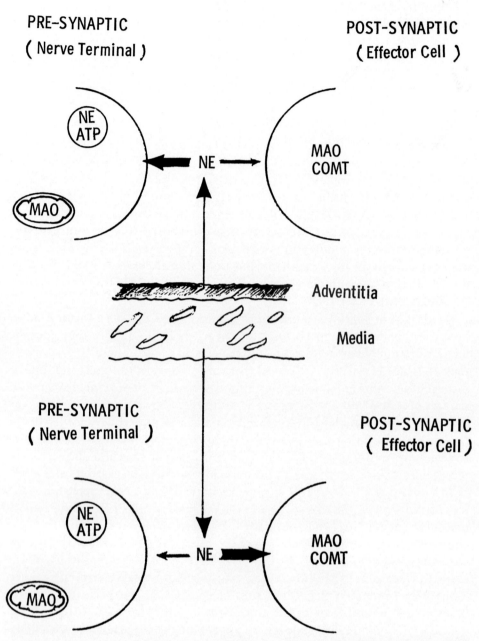

Figure 8. Schematic representation of inactivation of norepinephrine in vascular tissue. Adrenergic nerve terminals are distributed only in adventia and the underlying portion of the media of the blood vessels and aorta. Therefore, in this portion of the blood vessel, norepinephrine is inactivated by uptake into the nerve endings. Metabolism of norepinephrine by MAO and COMT occurs to a relatively small extent. In the greater part of the media, on the other hand, norepinephrine is inactivated solely by enzymatic metabolism. The potentiating action of cocaine is therefore largely confined to the adventitia.

inactivation by binding seems to predominate over inactivation by enzymatic destruction, whereas in the greater part of the media norepinephrine is inactivated not by uptake but primarily by enzymatic breakdown.

EXTRANEURONAL UPTAKE

When the organ is denervated either by surgical procedures or by administration of serum antinerve growth factor, there is a small uptake and retention of norepinephrine (Fischer *et al.*, 1965; Iverson *et al.*, 1966; Draskóczy and Trendelenburg, 1968).

Similarly, when the isolated guinea pig atria are incubated with ^{3}H-norepinephrine in the presence of cocaine, despite the inhibition of uptake of ^{3}H-catecholamine by cocaine, a small amount (10% to 20% of normal) of amine is retained. This store of norepinephrine is resistant to the releasing action of nicotine (Bhagat, Bovell and Robinson, 1967). Since in isolated guinea pig atria, the store from which nicotine releases catecholamine resembles the stores released by sympathetic nerve stimulation (Barnett and Benforado, 1966), it is conceivable that norepinephrine in this store cannot possibly be released by nerve impulses. The accumulation appears to occur outside of sympathetic neurons.

Similarly, when either isolated rat heart from a normal animal is perfused with norepinephrine in the presence of cocaine or isolated heart from an immunosympathectomized animal is perfused with norepinephrine, there is a small extraneuronal accumulation of norepinephrine (Eisenfeld, *et al.*, 1967a,b).

Histochemical studies of the rat heart after perfusion with high concentration of norepinephrine show a massive accumulation of unchanged catecholamine in cardiac muscle cells (Ehringer and Sporrong, 1968; Farnebo and Malmfors, 1969). Iversen (1965) referred to this uptake as uptake 2.

Extraneuronal accumulation also has been shown to occur in the arterial smooth muscle of cat's spleen (Gillespie and Hamilton, 1967), connective tissue (Avakin and Gillespie, 1968) and isolated nictitating membrane (Draskóczy and Trendelenburg, 1970).

Characteristics of Extraneuronal Uptake

Extraneuronal retention of norepinephrine is a transient phenomena. At least part of the extraneuronal norepinephrine leaves the stores without being metabolized. Therefore, it is likely that it then contributes to the concentration of amine at the receptors (Avakian and Gillespie, 1968; Draskózky and Trendelenburg, 1970). Extraneuronal accumulation of norepinephrine is reduced by adrenergic blocking agents. The alpha adrenergic blocking agents are more effective in this respect than beta-receptors blocking drugs. The adrenergic blocking agents reduce not only the extraneuronal ^{3}H-norepinephrine content but also the formation of o-methylated metabolite. Several other drugs, such as nylidrin, normetanephrine, metanephrine, synephrine, isoxusprine and various steroids, reduce the extra-neuronal accumulation of norepinephrine (Axelrod and Kopin, 1969).

There is a dissociation in the ability of the drugs to block the extra neuronal and intraneuronal uptake of norepinephrine. For example, meta-reminol, cocaine or reserpine inhibits the neuronal accumulation of norepi-nephrine but shows no effect on extraneuronal uptake and metabolism. On the other hand, normetanephrine, methoxyamine and steroids have a greater inhibitory effect on extraneuronal accumulation and metabolism of norepinephrine. The comparison of extraneuronal and intraneuronal uptake is summarized in Table III.

TABLE III
COMPARISON OF THE PROPERTIES OF NEURONAL AND
EXTRANEURONAL UPTAKE OF NOREPINEPHRINE

	NEURONAL	EXTRANEURONAL
BINDING	FIRM	RELATIVITY LESS FIRM
PHENOXYBENZAMINE	MARKED INHIBITION	MARKED INHIBITION
COCAINE	MARKED INHIBITION	NO EFFECT
NORMETANEPHRINE	SLIGHT INHIBITION	MARKED INHIBITION
METARAMINOL	MARKED INHIBITION	NO EFFECT
COLD	?	MARKED INHIBITION

Inhibition of COMT and MAO enhance the accumulation of extra-neuronal ^{3}H-norepinephrine (Draskoczy and Trendelenburg, 1970). There is a close relationship between extraneuronal uptake of norepinephrine and the activity of COMT. It appears that catecholamines and their o-meth-ylated metabolites compete for the same extraneuronal uptake or storage site(s). Thus, inhibition of COMT results in an increase in extraneuronal uptake of norepinephrine by decreasing the competition by o-methylated metabolites. Normetanephrine, by increasing the competition, reduces the extraneuronal uptake. The rates of extraneuronal uptake of amines are quite different from the relative rates of intraneuronal accumulation. Epi-nephrine, rather than norepinephrine, is a preferred amine for extraneuronal accumulation.

The Physiological Functions of Extraneuronal Uptake

The physiological significance of this extraneuronal uptake is not fully known, but it is unlikely that it has any major role in the inactivation process of released and circulating norepinephrine (Jonsson *et al.*, 1969). However, in many tissues in which the sympathetic innervation is only sparsely distributed in a large bulk of smooth muscles—for example, as in vascular smooth muscle—extraneuronal accumulation may play a role in the inactivation of released norepinephrine (Lightman and Iversen, 1969). This is supported by the fact that in such preparations, while inhibition of monoamine oxidase and catechol-o-methyl transferase may potentiate the response to norepinephrine and other amines (Kalsner and Nickerson, 1969), cocaine fails to do so (Maxwell *et al.*, 1966).

Since epinephrine rather than norepinephrine is the preferred substrate for extraneuronal uptake, it is possible that this system may have some role for the rapid removal of circulating epinephrine, which has been demonstrated in many perfused organs (Vane, 1969).

CHAPTER III

BIOSYNTHESIS OF CATECHOLAMINES

IN 1939 BLASCHKO proposed the biosynthetic pathway for catechol-amines which was finally established by Udenfriend and his co-workers (Nagatsu *et al.*, 1964). It proceeds as follows: 1-Tyrosine - - - Dopa - - - Dopamine - - - Norepinephrine - - - Epinephrine. The natural precursor for the synthesis of catecholamine is 1-tyrosine. The amount of the precursor, 1-tyrosine, present in the circulation is about 15 mg/liter. The adrenergic neuron receives the precursor from the blood. The nature and kinetics of tyrosine transport into the neuron are not known. Once inside the neuron, tyrosine is converted to dopa by the enzyme tyrosine hydroxylase (Nagatsu *et al.*, 1964). The enzyme is specific for 1-tyrosine and requires oxygen, iron and tetrahydropteridine cofactor for its activity. The enzyme is present in the brain (Iyer *et al.*, 1963; McGeer *et al.*, 1965), in the adrenal medulla and within the adrenergic nervous tissue. Its exact location in the neuron is not known. It does not seem to occur within the storage vesicles (Rutledge and Weiner, 1967; Musacchio, 1968). The relative low activity of this enzyme makes it the rate-limiting step in the biosynthesis of the catecholamines. In the neuronal cytoplasm, 1-dopa is decarboxylated to dopamine by the enzyme dopa decarboxylase, which is a soluble enzyme and is present in the cytoplasm of the neuron. Because of its wide substrate specificity and rela-tively very high activity, the enzyme does not play a significant role in regulating the synthesis of catecholamines. Dopamine formed from dopa is taken up into the storage particles where it is converted into norepineph-rine by the enzyme, dopamine-β-oxidase, which is a copper-containing enzyme and requires ascorbic acid and oxygen as co-factors (Levin and Kaufman, 1961). This enzyme is entirely localized in the storage granules, so that dopamine must enter the granules in order to be hydroxylated. This requirement is not necessary when the enzyme is solublized (Levin and Kaufman, 1961). Dopamine which is not taken up by the storage vesicle may be destroyed by monoamine oxidase. The norepinephrine forms a stable complex with ATP and protein in the vesicle. Norepinephrine which is not bound may leak into the cytoplasm and there may be deaminated by monoamine oxidase. The enzyme, dopamine-β-oxidase, is nonspecific and

THE BIOSYNTHESIS OF CATECHOLAMINES

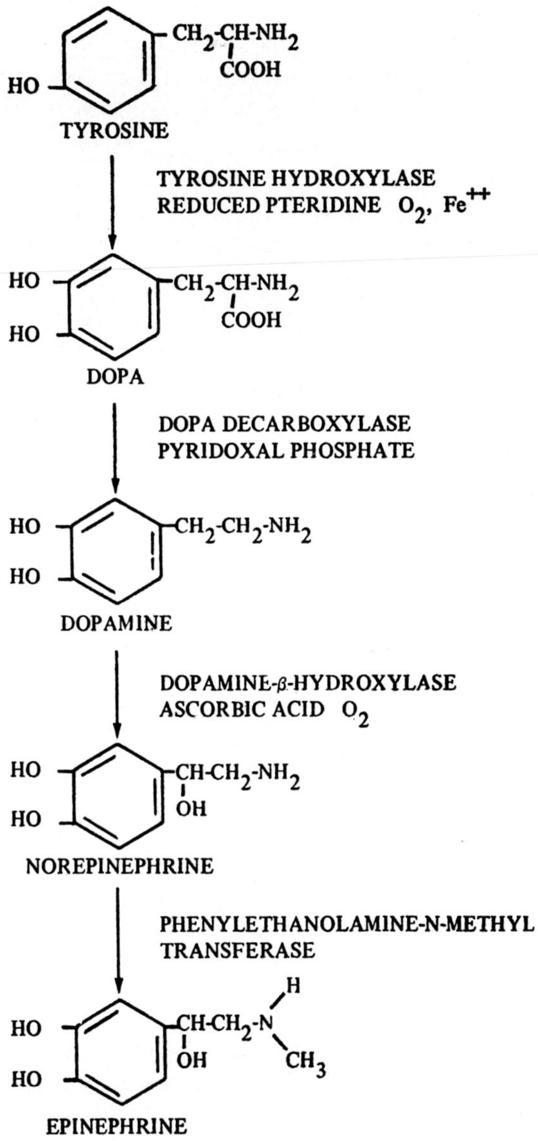

Figure 9.

can also β-hydroxylate other amines such as tyramine (Fischer *et al.*, 1964), β-phenylethylamine and α-methyl dopamine. Dopamine-β-oxidase enzyme is inhibited by treatment with disulfiram, which is reduced in the body to diethyldithiocarbamate. This inhibition results from chelation of the copper moiety of the dopamine-β-oxidase. Although this enzyme has a low activity compared to dopa decarboxylase, it is difficult to alter norepinephrine levels by inhibiting this enzyme.

The final step in the formation of catecholamine involves the N-methylation of norepinephrine. This conversion is catalyzed by phenylethanolamine-

N-methyl-transferase (PNMT) and occurs almost exclusively in the adrenal medulla, never in measurable amounts in nerves. The enzyme is found in the supernatant after high speed centrifugation and requires S-adenosyl methionine for transfer of the methyl group to the amino group of norepinephrine. It, (PNMT), is nonspecific and can methylate a variety of β-phenylethanolamines. The activity of this enzyme is controlled by glucocorticoids (Wurtman and Axelrod, 1966). In the absence of a glucocorticoid (Bhagat, *et al.*, 1971) as after hypophysectomy, the activity of the enzyme is reduced; restoration of glucocorticoids by dexamethasone activity of the enzymes returns to normal. In the adrenal medullary cell, norepinephrine migrates from chromaffin granules to the cytoplasm and is N-methylated to form epinephrine. Then epinephrine is also stored in the granules. The pathway in the biosynthesis of epinephrine is depicted in Figure 9.

RATE-LIMITING STEPS IN BIOSYNTHESIS OF NOREPINEPHRINE

The pharmacological inhibition of tyrosine hydroxylase or of dopamine β-oxidase decreases the rate of formation of norepinephrine. It has not yet been shown that the aromatic 1-amino acid decarboxylase can be inhibited to the point of interfering with catecholamine biosynthesis. In order to elucidate the rate-limiting enzyme, Levitt *et al.* (1965) compared the rate of formation of norepinephrine from three labelled precursors (tyrosine, dopa and dopamine) in isolated, perfused guinea pig heart. They found that the rate of norepinephrine synthesis in the isolated heart was greatly in excess of the normal *in vivo* rates. The rate of synthesis increased with increasing concentrations of labelled dopa or dopamine; maximal rates of synthesis, however, were not achieved even at concentrations approaching $10^{-3}M$. On the other hand, with labelled 1-tyrosine the maximal rate of synthesis of norepinephrine was achieved at a concentration below $10^{-4}M$. This is consistent with a measured K_m of about $10^{-5}M$ for purified tyrosine hydroxylase (Ikeda *et al.*, 1965). The activity of tyrosine hydroxylase is always much lower than that of dopa decarboxylase or dopamine β-oxidase in tissue extract. For example, in the adrenal medulla, tyrosine hydroxylase activity is about 1000 times less than that of other synthetic enzymes. Furthermore, inhibition of this enzyme by α-methyl-p-tyrosine causes reduction in tissue endogenous catecholamine levels. On the basis of these observations, Levitt *et al.* (1965) concluded that tyrosine hydroxylase is the rate-limiting enzyme.

Although the maximum rate of catecholamine synthesis is limited by the capacity of tyrosine hydroxylase to convert tyrosine to dopa, it is still an oversimplification to consider tyrosine hydroxylase as the only controlling step in catecholamine synthesis.

Dopamine formed in the axoplasm of the neuron is taken up by the storage vesicles or is deaminated by monoamine oxidase present in large amounts in the neuron. With uptake into the granule β-hydroxylation must therefore be a second site at which catecholamine synthesis can be regulated.

Furthermore, several procedures which cause induction of tyrosine hydroxylase can increase the levels of dopamine β-hydroxylase.

REGULATION OF SYNTHESIS OF NOREPINEPHRINE

Physiological factors which control the rate of synthesis of norepinephrine in the adrenergic neurons are complex. Since endogenous levels of norepinephrine are maintained at a fixed level characteristic of each organ unless synthesis is inhibited, it appears that there is a dynamic balance between the rates of synthesis of norepinephrine and its disappearance.

Regulation of Synthesis Through End-Product Inhibition

When the splanchnic nerves to the adrenal medulla are stimulated, there is a large increase in the catecholamine content of the venous effluent; but there is little or no reduction in the catecholamine content of the medullary tissue. Bhagat (1967) showed that increased sympathetic nervous activity produced by: 1) sympathetic nerve stimulation for 1 hour; 2) exposure to cold for 6 hours; or 3) administration of drugs like histamine and β-tetrahydronaphthylamine, causes little change in cardiac catecholamine levels. The maintenance of the endogenous amine level is not possible, however, when norepinephrine synthesis is inhibited by the tyrosine hydroxylase inhibitor, α-methyl-tyrosine. In this case catecholamine content is reduced significantly. Thus, these findings suggest that catecholamine synthesis is, indeed, increased in response to sympathetic nerve stimulation to maintain normal levels of catecholamines in the organ. Exposure to cold results in increased sympathetic nervous activity and release of catecholamines. When rats were exposed to 4° C for 3 hours there was a significant release of ^{3}H-norepinephrine, whereas the endogenous cardiac catecholamine remained unaltered. Thus, the relative stability of endogenous norepinephrine in tissue during high impulse activity associated with cold exposure, accompanied by a release of ^{3}H-norepinephrine, indicates the increase in rate of synthesis of catecholamines. Estimates of norepinephrine synthesis from the slopes of decline in specific activity of norepinephrine with time (Brodie *et al.*, 1966), showed a four-fold increase in the rate of synthesis of norepinephrine. The increase in synthesis of norepinephrine induced by nerve stimulation also has been demonstrated in the heart (Oliverio and Stjärne, 1965; Gorden *et al.*, 1966a, b; Bhagat, 1969c), brain (Bhagat, 1969a, b; 1970), and submandibular gland (Sedvall and Kopin, 1967a). It has also been demonstrated in the isolated adrenal gland and in the isolated guinea-pig vas deferens (Weiner and Alouis, 1966).

Acceleration of norepinephrine synthesis due to nerve stimulation occurs at the tyrosine hydroxylation step because the rate of formation of ^{3}H-norepinephrine, from dopa-^{3}H and dopamine-^{3}H, remains unaltered during nerve stimulation (Sedvall and Kopin, 1967b; Dairman *et al.*, 1968).

Recently, Weiner and Rabadjija (1968a, b) have shown that when vasa

deferentia of guinea pig, set up in an organ bath, were incubated with
³H-tyrosine for one hour the uptake of ³H-tyrosine and its incorporation
into the protein of each are similar in both stimulated and unstimulated
preparations. The formation of ³H-norepinephrine from ³H-tyrosine was
inhibited in the vas deferens preparation in the presence of $1\mu g/ml$ of
norepinephrine. This exogenous norepinephrine also blocked the accelerated synthesis of norepinephrine which is ordinarily seen during nerve
stimulation.

A small fraction of the noradrenaline which is outside the vesicles in
the axoplasm may be the critical compound for the regulation of tyrosine
hydroxylase. Alternatively, dopamine, normally found outside of the vesicle,
may be responsible for regulating tyrosine hydroxylase activity. Release of
endogenous norepinephrine may increase the free intraneuronal norepine-
nephrine in the cytoplasm and block its own synthesis. Stimulation may, in
some way, reduce the free cytoplasmic catecholamine concentration and
thereby activate the tyrosine hydroxylase and increase the rate of synthesis.
Inhibition of monoamine oxidase would preserve the free intraneuronal
norepinephrine and thus, may lead to an inhibition of norepinephrine
synthesis. Neff and Costa (1966) have shown that pargyline (a monoamine
oxidase inhibitor) inhibits the turnover rate of norepinephrine. The
synthesis of cardiac norepinephrine is not changed immediately after the
injection of MAO inhibitor, when the catecholamine levels are not yet
increased, even though MAO is almost completely blocked (Ngai *et al.*,
1968).

Since a decrease in an inhibitory end-product, i.e. norepinephrine, seems
to be responsible for the enhanced norepinephrine synthesis during increase
in sympathetic nerve activity, there is no necessity for an increase in enzyme
protein. Thus, procedures which modify directly or indirectly the rate of
metabolism of norepinephrine may indirectly affect the rate of synthesis
of norepinephrine. This mechanism is capable of rapidly adjusting the rate of
synthesis by altering the activity of tyrosine hydroxylase without changing
the actual level of enzyme. This probably accounts for the bulk of regulation necesary to maintain the homeostasis.

Increase in Norepinephrine Synthesis in Poststimulation Period

The increased norepinephrine synthesis occurs both during the period of
nerve stimulation and in the poststimulation period. Weiner and Rabadjija
(1968c) have shown that, in isolated nerve vas deferens preparation, the
synthesis of ¹⁴C-catecholamine from ¹⁴C-tyrosine is increased not only during
interval stimulation at a rate of 30/sec for 60 minutes, but also in the poststimulation period. The mechanism involved in the acceleration of norepinephrine synthesis during and after stimulation seems to be distinct.
While exogenous norepinephrine is able to inhibit partially or to abolish
the accelerated norepinephrine synthesis seen during nerve stimulation, it
does not affect the increased norepinephrine synthesis demonstrable in the

poststimulation period. Accelerated norepinephrine synthesis during the period of stimulation is not abolished by puromycin, a potent inhibitor of protein synthesis, whereas the accelerated synthesis in the poststimulation period is not seen when protein synthesis is inhibited by this agent (Weiner and Rabadjija, 1968c).

The exact mechanism of this increase in rate of synthesis during post-stimulation has not been elucidated as yet; it appears that it could be due to an altered substrate availability or changes in end-product inhibition. It is not due to an increase in tyrosine hydroxylase content since an increase in tyrosine hydroxylase activity under similar experimental conditions was not found.

Increase in Rate of Synthesis of Norepinephrine Through Increased Enzyme Synthesis

When the increase in the sympathetic nervous activity is maintained for a prolonged period of time, it provokes a long term adaptation which involves the induction of tyrosine hydroxylase. This increase in content of tyrosine hydroxylase can be produced by a wide variety of pharmacological and other stimuli.

Recently, Axelrod and his co-workers (Mueller *et al.*, 1969a, b; Thoenen *et al.*, 1969a, b) have found that pretreatment of rats with reserpine, 6-hydroxydopamine or phenoxybenzamine caused an increase in the tyrosine hydroxylase activity in the adrenal glands, sympathetic ganglia and brain stem. All of the above drugs interfere with postganglionic sympathetic transmission by different mechanisms.

Reserpine depletes norepinephrine from its stores in the postganglionic sympathetic nerve ending and thereby reduces the sympathetic nerve activity. Administration of 6-hydroxydopamine causes degeneration of adrenergic axon terminal (Tranzer and Thoenen, 1967; 1968). The other parts of adrenergic neuron, its cell body and other tissue structure, particularly cholinergic nerve endings, are left unaffected by this treatment (Thoenen and Tanzer, 1968a, b); thus, its treatment causes chemical sympathectomy. Phenoxybenzamine makes neurotransmitters ineffective at receptor sites by occupying the receptive site. All these procedures cause an activation of compensatory mechanisms resulting in an increase in the activity of the sympatho-adrenal system. This increase in the rate of synthesis of norepinephrine is preceded by an increase in tyrosine hydroxylase activity. De Quattro *et al.* (1969) have shown that in the rabbit made hypertensive by chronic denervation of the carotid sinuses and aortic arch, the tyrosine hydroxylase activity in the myocardium increased. Bhagat (unpublished) has found an increase in cardiac tyrosine hydroxylase activity in rats, 24 days after demedullation of adrenal glands. Recently, Van Woert and Korb (1970) determined the effect of total body x-irradiation, another stress producing agent, on catecholamine and tyrosine hydroxylase levels. They found an increase in adrenal tyrosine hydroxylase activity when measured at 72 and 84 hours. Thus, these observations suggest that when an increase in the sympathetic impulse traffic is maintained for a longer period, there is an increase in synthesis of tyrosine hydroxylase and an increased content of this enzyme in adrenergic nervous tissue. This increase in tyrosine hydroxylase must be responsible for enhanced synthesis of norephinephrine observed.

Increased enzyme activity is due to the formation of new enzyme molecules, since inhibition of protein synthesis with either cyclohexamide or actinomycin prevents the drug-induced increase of tyrosine hydroxylase in the adrenal gland and in sympathetic ganglion (Mueller *et al.*, 1969a, b).

This increased enzyme production and activity induced by prolonged stimulation of sympathetic nervous system can be antagonized by prior decentralization (Thoenen *et al.*, 1969a, b), by ganglionic blocking agents or by preganglionic denervation. These results suggest that an increased enzyme activity follows chronic increase in tonic impulse traffic.

Increased sympathetic nerve activity over a period of days results not only in elevation of tyrosine hydroxylase but also dopamine β-hydroxylase (Axelrod, 1972) in the adrenal gland, sympathetic nerve terminals and nerve cell bodies. Phenylethanolamine-N-methyltransferase (PNMT), another enzyme involved in the biosynthesis of catecholamines, converts norepinephrine to epinephrine. Increase in PNMT in adrenal gland also occurs by procedures which cause induction of tyrosine hydroxylase and dopamine β-oxidase. The temporal aspects of these changes are, however, different for the tyrosine hydroxylase and PNMT. Tyrosine hydroxylase activity increased 12 to 18 hours after reserpine while that of PNMT was only elevated 30 hours after administration of reserpine (Bhagat *et al.*, 1971).

Hormones have also been found to influence the catecholamine biosynthetic enzymes in the adrenal gland. Removal of the pituitary gland results in a gradual but marked reduction in activities of tyrosine hydroxylase, dopamine-β-hydroxylase, and phenylethanolamine-N-methyltransferase. Activity of all these enzymes in hypophysectomized animals can be restored by repeated administration of adrenocorticotropic hormone (ACTH). The potent corticoid dexamethasone restores the activity of PNMT, but not that of tyrosine hydroxylase. Thus, chronic increase in sympathetic adrenal activity elevates the activities of tyrosine hydroxylase, dopamine-β-hydroxylase and PNMT in the adrenal medulla. The increase in tyrosine hydroxylase activity is due mainly to neural activity, that of dopamine-β-hydroxylase is due to both nerve activity and ACTH, and PNMT activity is elevated mainly by humoral factors (Axelrod and Weinshelboum, 1972).

SUMMARY

Two mechanisms seem to control catecholamine synthesis, one involving end-product inhibition of tyrosine hydroxylase and the other involving enzyme induction. Regulation of synthesis by end-product inhibition is rapid and the rate of synthesis of norepinephrine is adjusted immediately in response to changes in physiological demands for catecholamine. It is usually believed that only the intraneuronally unbound catecholamine is important in the feedback control of norepinephrine synthesis. An increase in sympathetic nerve activity, due to any stimulus, would increase the efflux of norepinephrine, and thereby could lower slightly the free intraneuronal cytoplasmic levels of the neurohormone. This decrease might diminish the end-product inhibition, and thereby stimulate norepinephrine synthesis. On the other hand, procedures which either decrease the efflux of norepinephrine or which release norepinephrine from storage vesicles into cytoplasm, elicit an increase in free intraneuronal catecholamine and consequently an end-product inhibition of tyrosine hydroxylase occurs; this would exert an inhibitory effect on norepinephrine synthesis. It probably accounts for most of the regulation necessary to maintain the homeostasis.

The other mechanism, (i.e. enzyme induction) of control of norepinephrine synthesis, becomes effective only as a result of prolonged stimulation of the sympathetic nervous system. In this case, an increase in the rate of synthesis of norepinephrine is due to an increase in the synthesis and content of tyrosine hydroxylase. This process, however, is relatively slower.

CHAPTER IV

FALSE NEUROTRANSMITTERS

WHILE NOREPINEPHRINE IS a neurochemical transmitter of the sympathetic nervous system in mammals, a number of sympatho-mimetic amines, chemically related to norepinephrine, behave like these catecholamines. Following administration, these amines, such as α-methyl norepinephrine and metaraminol, are taken up by sympathetic nerve endings and may replace the norepinephrine from its storage site (s). These amines can be released by sympathetic nerve stimulation and by reserpine, guanethidine and tyramine, all of which deplete norepinephrine. The uptake of these amines is inhibited by drugs inhibiting norepinephrine uptake. Thus, these amines act as "false neurotransmitters" (Kopin, 1966).

SYNTHESIS OF FALSE NEUROTRANSMITTERS

The processes responsible for synthesis, storage and release of norepine-phrine are not entirely specific. Structurally related compounds may be formed also, stored in sympathetic nerve terminals in the granules, and may be released by sympathetic impulses. Out of the three enzymes responsible for formation of norepinephrine from tyrosine, only the first enzyme, tyro-sine hydroxylase, is relatively specific. The other two enzymes, dopa de-carboxylase and dopamine β-oxidase are relatively non-specific.

Several amino acids, such as α-methyl dopa and α-methyl-m-tyrosine, initially used as inhibitors of dopa-decarboxylase, but were subsequently found to deplete norepinephrine by different mechanisms (Udenfriend et al., 1962). It was found that these synthetic amino acids can be de-carboxylated by dopa decarboxylase and subsequently taken up by granular vesicles which contain dopamine β-oxidase. In the storage vesicles they are β-hydroxylated (Fig. 10).

The β-hydroxylated compounds, α-methyl norepinephrine or metaraminol, are accumulated in the adrenergic neuron (Carlsson and Lindquist, 1962; Day and Rand, 1964; Crout and Shore, 1964; Crout et al., 1964). In the body, tyrosine is partly decarboxylated to form tyramine, but normally tyramine is readily destroyed by monoamine oxidase. When monoamine oxidase is inhibited, it leads to accumulation of tyramine in the sympathetic

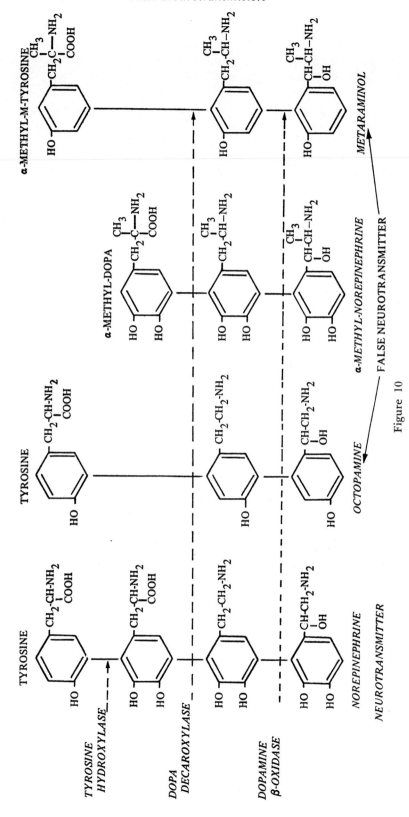

Figure 10

nerves and is β-hydroxylated in granules to octopamine (Kopin, *et al.*, 1965). Similarly when α-methyl-tyramine-^{3}H, which is not a substrate for monoamine oxidase, is administered, α-methyl octopamine appears in the cardiac tissue (Kopin *et al.*, 1964).

Effect of False Neurotransmitters on Synthesis of Norepinephrine

There are three possible effects of a false neurotransmitter on synthesis of norepinephrine. First, false transmitters that have catechols may compete with the tetrahydropteridine cofactor for the reduced enzyme and inhibit the conversion of tyrosine to dopa, resulting in a diminished synthesis. Second, the false transmitter may compete with dopamine for the site of its synthesis, so that less dopamine will be converted to norepinephrine. Finally, the false transmitter may displace the norepinephrine from its storage site into the cytoplasm, resulting in increased free intraneuronal norepinephrine and consequent end-product feedback inhibition of tyrosine hydroxylase. Kopin *et al.* (1969) have shown that the accumulation of false transmitter in the rat heart is accompanied by a diminished synthesis of norepinephrine. On the other hand, when octopamine is rapidly removed, norepinephrine synthesis is accelerated.

Effect of False Transmitter on the Release of Norepinephrine

False transmitter replaces the norepinephrine from its storage site on a

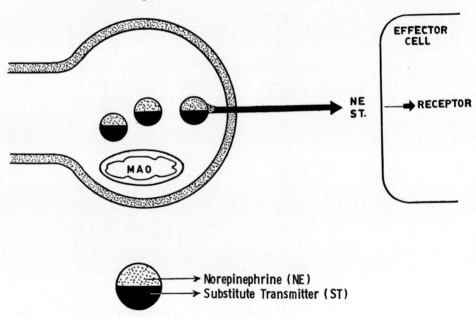

Figure 11. *Diagrammatic illustration of transmitter released in the presence of a substitute transmitter.* Foreign amine derived from α-Methyl Dopa and α-Methyl-M-Tyrosine may replace Norepinephrine in the storage vesicles and act as a false transmitter. Replacement of Norepinephrine by a substitute transmitter results in a diminished release of Norepinephrine and therefore apparent adrenergic blockade.

mole-for-mole basis. If a nerve impulse releases a certain number of molecules, the presence of a substitute may diminish the quantity of physiological transmitter released (Fig. 11).

Effect on the Uptake of Norepinephrine

By competing for the neuronal uptake of norepinephrine, false transmitter can reduce the uptake of norepinephrine, resulting in the potentiation of the effect of the released norepinephrine. Bhagat and Ragland (1966) have shown that low doses of metaraminol (0.02 mg/kg) cause an increase in sensitivity of the blood pressure of the reserpine pretreated cat to norepinephrine, presumably by blocking its uptake into the nerve terminal. In high doses (1 mg/kg), metaraminol causes subsensitivity of the blood-pressure response of reserpine-pretreated cats to norepinephrine. This effect could be due to occupation of the receptors by metaraminol, thus limiting the number of available receptor sites for activation by the administered norepinephrine.

PHYSIOLOGICAL CONSEQUENCE OF ACCUMULATION OF FALSE TRANSMITTER

The functional consequence of norepinephrine depletion by α-methylnorepinephrine may differ greatly from that observed after administration of reserpine and guanethidine. There is not only a loss of transmitter as in the case of reserpine and guanethidine but instead, a replacement of the part of the transmitter by α-methyl norepinephrine. This can take over its function and act as a false neurotransmitter. However, at the receptor's site, it may exert weaker action than the natural transmitter, norepinephrine, and hereby diminish the effect of sympathetic stimulation. This mechanism may explain, at least in part, the antihypertensive effect of α-methyl dopa. The formation of false transmitter, octopamine, in the adrenergic nerve also has been suggested to account for the sympathetic blockade and hypotension in man after long-term administration of MAO inhibitors, such as pargyline.

CHAPTER V

SUMMARY OF THE EVENTS AT ADRENERGIC

NEUROEFFECTOR ORGANS

1. Synthesis of Norepinephrine

a. Synthesis of norepinephrine takes place from tyrosine within the sympathetic neurons. It involves three enzymatically catalyzed chemical reactions.

b. The synthetic precursor, 1-tyrosine, normally present in the circulation about 15 mg/L) enters the axonal membrane by a concentrating mechanism. The kinetics of tyrosine transport into adrenergic neurons are not known.

c. It is then hydroxylated to dopa by tyrosine hydroxylase, the rate-limiting enzyme in norepinephrine synthesis. The exact intracellular location of this reaction is not known.

d. The resulting dopamine then enters the granulated storage vesicles which exhibit characteristic dense core.

e. It is β-hydroxylated to norepinephrine, by the enzyme dopamine β-oxidase present. Alternate biosynthetic pathways also exist.

f. Some of the dopamine is oxidatively deaminated by monoamine oxidase before it is taken up into the storage vesicles.

2. Storage Vesicles

a. These intracellular vesicles or granules are located mostly in varicosities at sympathetic nerve endings. These granules are synthesized in the cell bodies and transported at a rate of several millimeters per hour down the axon to the varicosities of the nerve terminals. The granules contain ATP and protein which may form a storage complex with norepinephrine (ratio 1:4).

3. Binding and Storage of Norepinephrine

a. The binding of norepinephrine by these granules prevents oxidation of the amine by intracellular monoamine oxidase (MAO).

b. The newly synthesized norepinephrine remains in unbound form for a short period and may be preferentially released.

c. The binding sites in granules are not entirely specific for norepinephrine. The compound structurally related to norepinephrine can also be retained by these vesicles.

d. Norepinephrine leaving the granules and entering the cytoplasm is mainly oxidatively deaminated by MAO in mitochondria.

e. After inhibition of MAO the released norepinephrine is taken up and stored again, resulting in elevation of tissue levels of catecholamine. Thus, intraneuronal MAO plays an important role in the regulation of endogenous amine levels.

4. Release of Norepinephrine

a. When the impulses, traveling down the nerve fiber, invade the nerve terminal, a sequence of events is initiated which terminates in a release of a transmitter. Calcium ions are required for this event.

b. Norepinephrine that is released passes into the space between the nerve and the muscle (synaptic cleft).

c. This norepinephrine diffuses across the gap to the smooth muscle where a small portion of it combines with a specialized part of the membrane called the receptor.

d. A consequence of this transmitter receptor interaction is a change in the activity of the cell and the biological response of the tissue.

e. A fraction of released norepinephrine is O-methylated by catechol-O-methyl transferase or diffused into the circulation from the extracellular space. This diffused norepinephrine is ultimately metabolized in the liver by COMT. The major fraction is taken up by the nerves and bound again into the granules.

f. Thus, the physiological importance of norepinephrine re-uptake may consist not only in termination of the action of released norepinephrine on the receptors, but also in conservation of the sympathetic transmitter.

g. In addition to synthesis, this process of reincorporation plays an important role for maintaining the levels of neurotransmitter amine at adrenergic neuron terminals constant.

5. Control of Synthesis or Norepinephrine

a. The rate of synthesis of norepinephrine depends upon various known and unknown factors.

b. The rate of conversion of tyrosine to norepinephrine is increased in response to nerve stimulation both *in vivo* and *in vitro*.

c. The rate of conversion of dopa to norepinephrine during nerve stimulation remains unaltered.

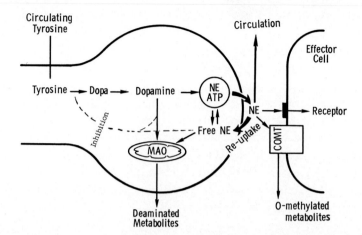

Figure 12. A diagrammatic representation of adrenergic nerve endings. Tyrosine is taken up into the neuron where it is converted to dopa by means of the enzyme tyrosine hydroxylase. Dopa is decarboxylated to dopamine by dopa decarboxylase. Dopamine is taken up by granular vesicles where it is converted to norepinephrine by means of the enzyme dopamine β-hydroxylase. Reserpine interferes with the uptake of dopamine into its site of synthesis. Norepinephrine is bound within the dense core vesicle, presumably to ATP and protein to form a stable complex. Norepinephrine which is not bound is released into the cytoplasm. The levels of free catecholamines in the intraneuronal cytoplasm regulate the rate of synthesis of norepinephrine by a negative feedback mechanism. Norepinephrine which is released into the cytoplasm is mostly exposed to the action of monoamine oxidase. Norepinephrine which is released into the synaptic cleft is partly exposed to catechol-o-methyl transferase, while another part is reincorporated into the stores and the remainder diffuses away from the site of liberation. A very small amount exerts its action on receptors.

    d. During nerve stimulation the levels of tyrosine hydroxylase in the tissues remain constant.

    e. Thus, acceleration is not a consequence of synthesis of more tyrosine hydroxylase.

    f. It is suggested that free intraneuronal norepinephrine inhibits the norepinephrine synthesis by negative feedback inhibition of tyrosine hydroxylase.

    g. Stimulation in some way may reduce the intraneuronal norepinephrine concentration at the enzyme site, and would release the tyrosine hydroxylase from end product inhibition.

    h. Inhibition of monoamine would preserve the intraneuronal norepinephrine and thus inhibit the synthesis of norepinephrine.

    i. The rapid regulation of catecholamine synthesis appears to be due to a release of tyrosine hydroxylase from the end-product inhibition.

    j. The enhanced synthesis occurs not only during nerve stimulation but also during the poststimulation period.

    k. This increase in synthesis in the poststimulation period is inhibited by puromycin.

l. There is no change in tyrosine hydroxylase enzyme activity during the period immediately following stimulation.

m. The exact mechanism for this increase of rate of synthesis of norepinephrine is yet to be determined.

n. Drugs which block the storage, or increase the release of norepinephrine from the axon into the cytoplasm will inhibit the synthesis of norepinephrine.

o. Tissue tyrosine hydroxylase levels are significantly increased when sympathetic nervous activity remains increased for a more prolonged period.

p. Several procedures, either surgical or chemical, which cause an increase in sympathetic nervous activity for a prolonged period produce an increase in the tyrosine hydroxylase content in the tissue.

q. The time to produce an increase in enzyme levels varies with the intensity of the stimulus employed.

r. Thus, catecholamine synthesis is regulated by two mechanisms: one involving end-product inhibition and the other by increasing the enzyme synthesis.

6. Uptake and Binding of Exogenous Norepinephrine

a. When norepinephrine is administered or infused, it is rapidly removed from the blood, half by tissue uptake and half by enzymatic inactivation.

b. Uptake and binding in various tissues is accomplished by sympathetic nerves which supply the tissue and serve to inactivate the hormones, protect them from degradation and store them for future re-use.

c. This inactivation by binding seems to dominate over inactivation by metabolism.

d. Compounds like cocaine, imipramine and chlorpromazine interfere with the uptake of norepinephrine into the nerve terminals, cause supersensitivity to norepinephrine because norepinephrine may reach higher concentrations at the receptors of the effector organs.

e. This uptake is saturable temperature dependent, requires sodium ion, and selective for the physiologically active l-isomers of norepinephrine and epinephrine.

f. Norepinephrine appears to be transported across the cell membrane more rapidly than epinephrine.

g. The retention of exogenous norepinephrine may be regarded as a combination of two steps, actual uptake into the nerve terminal followed by storage in vesicles.

h. Pretreatment with reserpine leaves the first step intact, but prevents the second. Thus, in reserpine pretreated animals, norepinephrine is transported at a normal rate, but instead of being stored in vesicle it is inactivated enzymatically by monoamine oxidase.

7. Metabolism of Infused Norepinephrine

a. Metabolic transformation takes place in most tissues. The major pathway of metabolic inactivation is first O-methylation to the 3-methoxy-derivatives, metanephrine and normetanephrine, by action of catechol-O-methyl transferase, and then deamination by action of monoamine oxidase. A major end-product is 3-methoxyl-4-hydroxymandelic acid (vanillylmandelic acid, VMA). Nearly complete metabolic transformation occurs, and of the various end products excreted in the urine, VMA and the metanephrines account for most.

b. Denervation experiments indicate that MAO is localized both within the neuron and outside the neuron while catechol-O-methyl transferase is present mainly outside the neuron.

c. The role of MAO and COMT in the destruction and inactivation of catecholamines is complicated. It varies with the tissues and the species. It also depends on whether the norepinephrine is circulating or bound.

d. Monoamine oxidase does not play a major role in terminating the activity of circulating catecholamine, it is largely responsible for intraneuronal destruction of norepinephrine and thereby regulates the levels of norepinephrine in the tissue.

e. Catechol-O-methyl transferase acts on extraneuronal norepinephrine and circulating norepinephrine.

f. Inactivation by metabolism is less important than inactivation by binding, since physiological effects of injected norepinephrine are rapidly terminated even after both monoamine oxidase and catechol-O-methyl transferase are inhibited.

SECTION TWO

THE
CARDIOVASCULAR SYSTEM

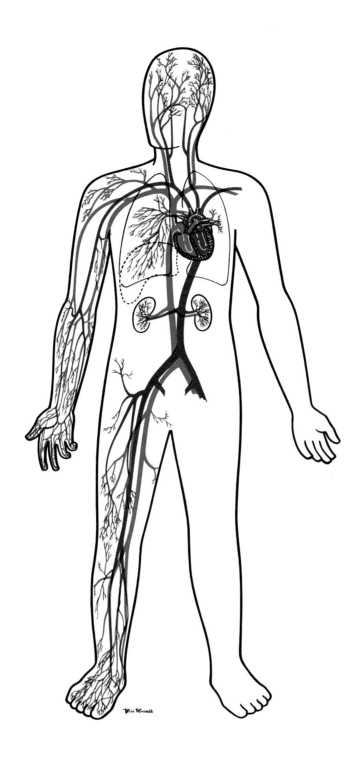

A **The Circulatory System**

Plate 1 A Diagram reprinted with permission of the American Heart Association.

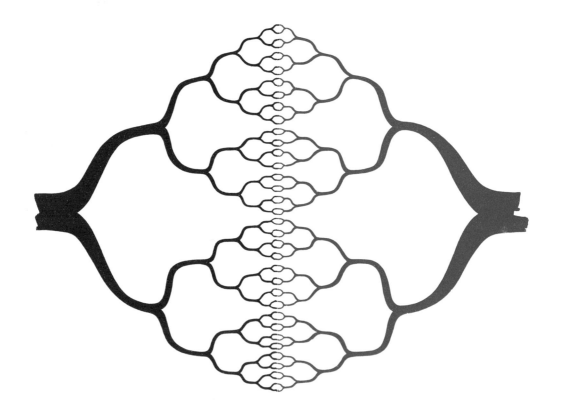

ARTERY - CAPILLARY - VEIN
SEQUENCE: (systemic circulation)

Blood flows from
arteries to veins

B

Plate 1 B

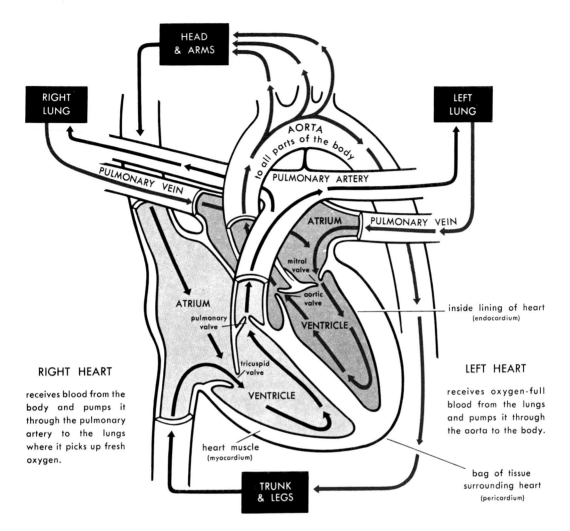

HEAD & ARMS

RIGHT LUNG

LEFT LUNG

AORTA

to all parts of the body

PULMONARY VEIN

PULMONARY ARTERY

ATRIUM

PULMONARY VEIN

mitral valve

aortic valve

ATRIUM

pulmonary valve

VENTRICLE

inside lining of heart (endocardium)

tricuspid valve

RIGHT HEART

receives blood from the body and pumps it through the pulmonary artery to the lungs where it picks up fresh oxygen.

VENTRICLE

heart muscle (myocardium)

LEFT HEART

receives oxygen-full blood from the lungs and pumps it through the aorta to the body.

bag of tissue surrounding heart (pericardium)

TRUNK & LEGS

Plate 2 The heart weighs well under a pound and is only a little larger than the fist, but it is a powerful, long working, hard working organ. Its job is to pump blood to the lungs and to all the body tissues.

The heart is a hollow organ. Its tough, muscular wall (myocardium) is surrounded by a fiberlike bag (pericardium) and is lined by a thin, strong membrane (endocardium). A wall (septum) divides the heart cavity down the middle into a "right heart" and a "left heart". Each side of the heart is divided again into an upper chamber (called an atrium or auricle) and a lower chamber (ventricle). Valves regulate the flow of blood through the heart and to the pulmonary artery and the aorta.

The heart is really a double pump. One pump (the right heart) receives blood which has just come from the body after delivering nutrients and oxygen to the body tissues. It pumps this dark, bluish red blood to the lungs where the blood gets rid of a waste gas (carbon dioxide) and picks up a fresh supply of oxygen which turns it a bright red again. The second pump (the left heart) receives this "reconditioned" blood from the lungs and pumps it out through the great trunk-artery (aorta) to be distributed by smaller arteries to all parts of the body.

Diagram reprinted with permission of the American Heart Association.

CHAPTER VI

HEART

THE CARDIOVASCULAR SYSTEM (Plate 1 A & B) consists of (1) the heart, (2) the arteries, (3) the arterioles, (4) the capillaries, (5) the venules and (6) the veins (Fig. 13). The heart acts merely as a pump to circulate adequate blood through the tissues of the body.

Blood is considered as one of the connective tissues. It consists of cells suspended in a fluid matrix called plasma (Fig. 14). Its chief function is to supply oxygen and nutrients to the tissues for metabolism and to remove the products of that metabolism for excretion in the lungs and kidneys (Fig. 15). It also acts as a heat exchange medium for heat distribution and thereby maintains a stable temperature within the body under varying external conditions.

The various tissue circulations are arranged in parallel coupled circuits with certain morphologic and functional differentiation. These parallel-coupled circuits include the cerebral, coronary, renal, muscle, skin, bone, and splanchnic circulation; the most important components of the splanchnic circulation are the liver, the gastrointestinal tract, the spleen and the pancreas. This parallel circuit arrangement provides a means whereby blood flow to a tissue can vary independently of changes in blood pressure. (A general scheme of the circulatory system is shown in Fig. 16).

A working organ needs more nourishment and therefore a larger blood supply as compared to the resting organ. To cope with this situation the blood is shunted from the resting to the working organs. This is possible because the blood vessels are capable of selective constriction or dilatation.

In addition to such shifts of blood from inactive to active organs, the body has (comparable to the cardiac reserve) a reserve blood volume. In the resting state of the body all the blood is not in active circulation. Some of it is withdrawn and temporarily stored until there is a demand for it. The large veins of the abdomen and thorax and pulmonary veins may serve as reservoirs.

The flow of blood through the body is thus varied in the several parallel

45

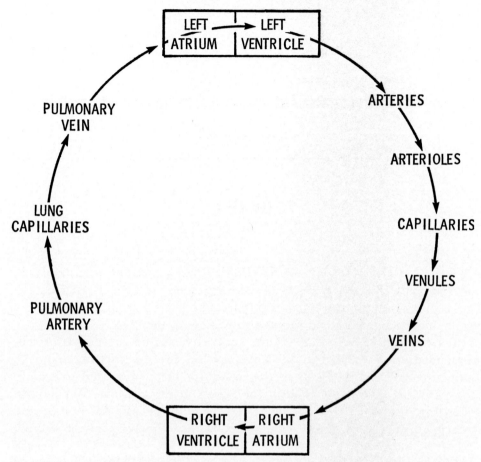

Figure 13. *Schematic representation of the flow of blood.* The left ventricle pumps the oxygenated blood through the aorta and arteries to the various tissue and organs of the body. Within each structure, blood flows from arteries to capillaries. It flows out of each organ through venules and then its veins to the right side of the heart. It is then pumped through the pulmonary artery to the lung arterioles and capillaries. In the lungs exchange of gases between blood and air takes place and venous blood is oxygenated. The oxygenated blood is returned to the left side of the heart via the four pulmonary veins.

circuits according to the specific biochemical needs of the particular organs. The heart and the blood vessel have been therefore provided with extensive control systems which serve to regulate tissue perfusion. Certain controls are intrinsic in the tissues of the heart and blood vessels, while additional control is provided by mechanisms that are extrinsic to the cardiovascular system (Fig. 17).

HEART

"The wisdom of the creator is seen in nothing more glorious than the heart". The heart is a specialized muscular tissue whose function is to contract periodically in order to pump adequate blood to meet the metabolic needs of the tissues of the body. It has a remarkable ability of adjusting

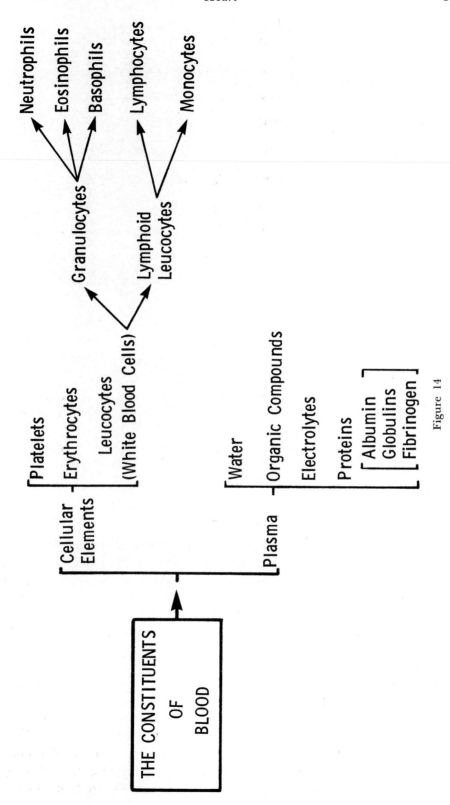

Figure 14

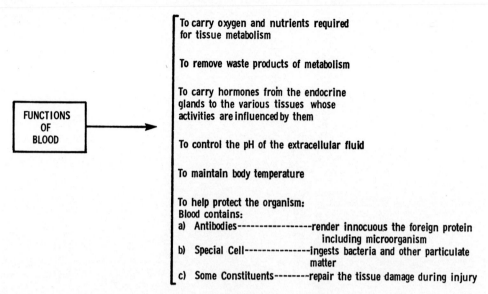

FUNCTIONS
OF
BLOOD

To carry oxygen and nutrients required
for tissue metabolism

To remove waste products of metabolism

To carry hormones from the endocrine
glands to the various tissues whose
activities are influenced by them

To control the pH of the extracellular fluid

To maintain body temperature

To help protect the organism:
Blood contains:
a) Antibodies----------------render innocuous the foreign protein
                                                   including microorganism
b) Special Cell--------------ingests bacteria and other particulate
                                              matter
c) Some Constituents--------repair the tissue damage during injury

Figure 15

its performance with ease and in a matter of seconds to meet the changing
conditions.

It contains four chambers: the right and left atria and the right and left
ventricles (Plate 2). The walls of each chamber consists of cardiac muscle
cells and the pumping action of the heart is a result of their contraction.
The atria are thin walled chambers whereas the ventricles are thicker
walled; the left ventricle is more muscular than the right because it has to
eject its blood into a high pressure system whereas the blood pressure on
the right ventricle is much lower.

HEART RATE

The heart beats according to its own inherent rhythm even in the absence
of any nervous or hormonal control. In normal resting adults, the heart
beats at a rate of 70 times per minute. The heart rate is significantly greater
in children. During sleep the heart rate diminishes by 10 to 20 beats per
minute, whereas during emotional excitment or muscular activity it may
increase to very high levels. In athletes at rest the heart rate is low. It is
usually 50 to 60 beats per minute. During swimming, heart rate decreases
in spite of the vigorous exercise of underwater swimming.

Superimposed on its own inherent rhythm is the tonic influence; the sino-
atrial node is under the tonic influence of both divisions of the autonomic
nervous system. The parasympathetic tone is predominant. The nervous
control of the heart rate has been elucidated by experimental studies on
animals. Stimulation of the vagus (or local application of acetylcholine to
the S.A. nodes) causes slowing of the heart whereas section of the vagus
nerves or administration of atropine elicit a pronounced tachycardia. In

GENERAL COURSE of the CIRCULATION

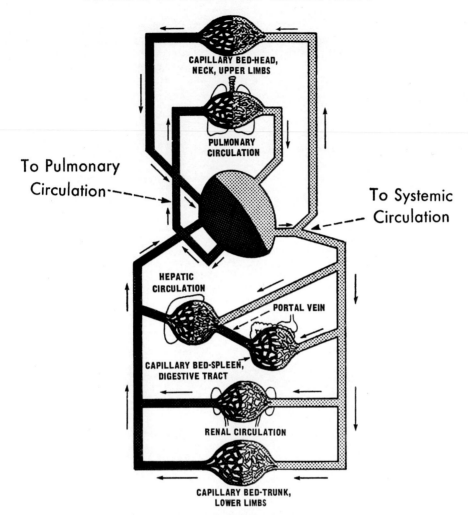

Figure 16. *Schematic representation of the circulatory system.* The cardiovascular system is divided into a number of parallel-coupled circuits with crtain morphologic and functional differentiation to supply the blood flow according to the metabolic requirements of the organs and tissues. This parallel circuit arrangement provides a means whereby blood flow to a tissue can vary independently of changes in blood pressure.

everyday activities there are several factors that can influence the heart rate. They include temperature, plasma electrolyte concentration, epinephrine, thyroxin, etc.

CONTRACTILITY OF THE HEART

As early as in 1914, Starling, a British physiologist, using a heart lung preparation studied the relationship between the diastolic volume and strength of contraction of the heart. He wrote "the law of the heart is the same as the law of initial length for skeletal muscle. The strength of con-

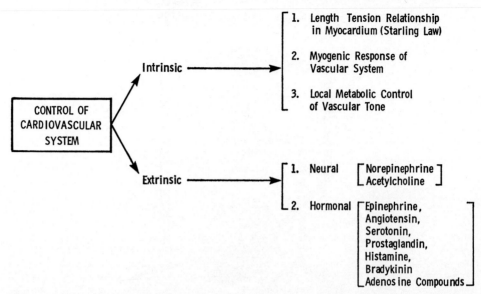

Figure 17. *Schematic representation of control systems regulating cardiovascular function.* Cardiovascular system is supplied with extensive control systems, some of which are intrinsic in the tissue of the myocardium and blood vessels, while others are extrinsic.

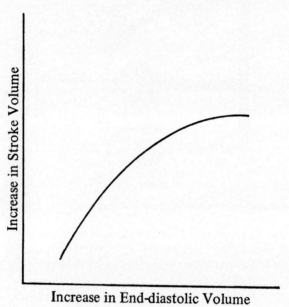

Figure 18. Simple diagram of Starling law of the heart. The stroke volume is plotted against end-diastolic volume. When the end-diastolic pressure increases above a certain point any further increase produces no or slight decrease in stroke volume.

traction is a function of muscle fiber length, i.e. stroke volume is directly proportional to diastolic filling". Thus he showed that the stroke output of the ventricle is primarily dependent on the filling pressure at the end of the diastolic, i.e. the higher the end-diastolic filling pressure the greater the

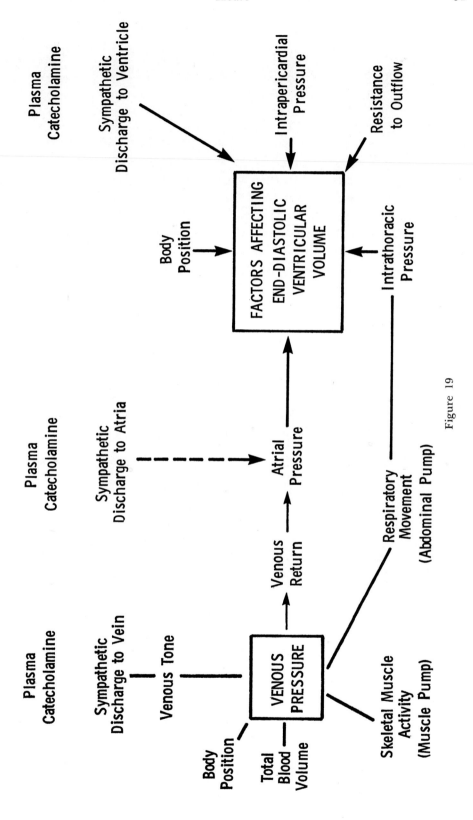

Figure 19

force of contraction. This gives a classic curve shown in Figure 18.

However, if the pressure is increased far enough the stroke output reaches a maximum and no longer responds to changes in filling pressure. The factors affecting the magnitude of ventricular end-diastolic volume are presented in Fig. 19. The intrinsic relationship between end-diastolic volume and stroke volume demonstrated in the heart lung preparation applies equally to intact human beings under resting conditions. It is an inherent, self regulatory mechanism by which heart muscle is able to adjust by changing end-diastolic volume; i.e. the heart will balance the stroke volume with the input. This law also has a role in balancing the outputs of the right and left ventricle in the normal animals. For example if the right ventricle pumps more blood than the left, the difference will cause an increase in the pulmonary venous pressure, which in turn will increase the diastolic filling of the left ventricle. The left ventricle will respond to this inherent mechanism by ejecting more blood, so correcting the right-left imbalance.

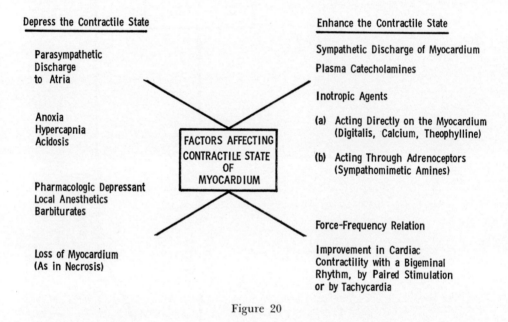

Depress the Contractile State

Parasympathetic
Discharge
to Atria

Anoxia
Hypercapnia
Acidosis

Pharmacologic Depressant
Local Anesthetics
Barbiturates

Loss of Myocardium
(As in Necrosis)

FACTORS AFFECTING
CONTRACTILE STATE
OF
MYOCARDIUM

Enhance the Contractile State

Sympathetic Discharge of Myocardium
Plasma Catecholamines

Inotropic Agents

(a) Acting Directly on the Myocardium
(Digitalis, Calcium, Theophylline)

(b) Acting Through Adrenoceptors
(Sympathomimetic Amines)

Force-Frequency Relation

Improvement in Cardiac
Contractility with a Bigeminal
Rhythm, by Paired Stimulation
or by Tachycardia

Figure 20

But this control mechanism is not the sole determinant of ventricular strength of contraction, since several factors can affect the level of ventricular performance, (Fig. 20). The most important factor is sympathetic nerves which can directly affect the ventricular function at any given level of end-diastolic volume or pressure. Starling himself recognized the importance of neurohormonal adjustments in adapting ventricular function to the body's requirement. In 1920 he wrote "No understanding of the circulatory reactions of the body is possible unless we start first with the fundamental properties of the heart muscle itself and then we find out how they are modified, protected and controlled under the influence of mechanisms—nervous, chemical, and mechanical—which under normal conditions play upon the heart".

Thus, stroke volume is controlled both by an intrinsic cardiac mechanism dependent only upon changes in end-diastolic volume and by an extrinsic mechanism mediated by the cardiac sympathetic nerves (and circulatory epinephrine).

INNERVATION OF THE HEART

Parasympathetic Pathway

Parasympathetic fibers originate in the medulla in the dorsal motor nucleus of the vagus. These fibers separate from the trunk of the nerve in the neck and intermingle with fibers of the sympathetic nerves to form the deep and superficial cardiac plexus and then continue on to innervate the atria. These fibers synapse with postganglionic cells located within the heart. Most of these ganglion cells are located in the sinoatrial (S.A.) node and atrioventricular (A.V.) conduction tissue. The right vagal nerve innervates the S.A. node and right atrium and produces slowing of the heart. The left vagal nerve innervates the A.V. conduction tissue and can cause heart block. There is no parasympathetic nerve supply to the ventricles (Fig. 21).

In laboratory experiments, stimulation of the vagus (Table IV) is known to cause:

1. Slowing of the heart
2. Prolongation of A.V. conduction time
3. Decrease in blood flow through the coronary artery
4. Complete ventricular arrest; (intense stimulation); if stimulation continues, the ventricle once again begins to contract, i.e. vagal escape occurs.
5. Decrease of atrial contractility and hence ventricular filling; it does not affect ventricular contractility. Tone in the heart is vagal in origin. Therefore, interruption of impulses along the vagus will increase the heart rate; (heart rate is often twice that of the initial rate).

Sympathetic Pathway

The sympathetic nerve originates in the medullary center, passes through the lateral column and synapses with the connector cell of the lateral horn of the grey matter. From the connector cells of the first four or five thoracic segments of the spinal cord, preganglionic fibers arise and synapse with postganglionic neurons located in the vertebral ganglia at the same level and in the inferior, middle and superior cervical ganglia. Postganglionic fibers from the right stellate ganglion supply principally the S-A node and the anterior wall of the ventricles; those from the left stellate ganglion supply mainly the A-V junction and the posterior wall of the ventricles (Fig. 21).

The organization of the cardiac sympathetic fibers is such that experimental stimulation of one stellate ganglion stimulates the whole myocardium, whereas stimulation of more peripheral parts of the nerves initiates a response only in a small area of myocardium.

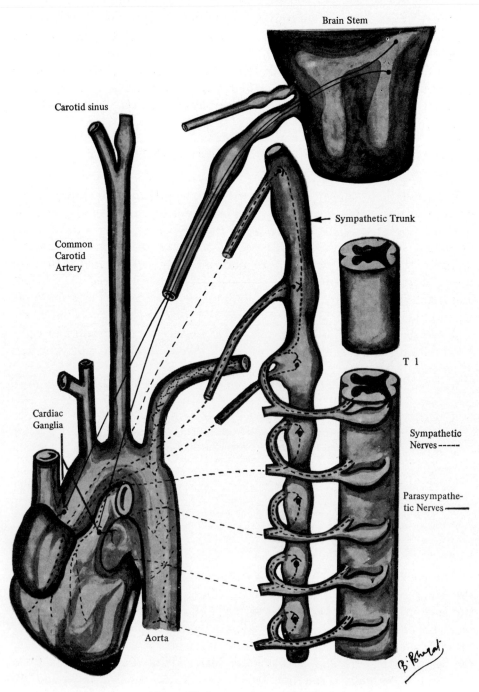

Figure 21. Innervation of the Heart.

FUNCTION OF THE SYMPATHETIC NERVOUS SYSTEM

Stimulation of a sympathetic nerve causes an increase in the rate of the heart beat and the force of its contraction and influences oxygen consumption and coronary blood flow (Table IV). There is also an increase in sympathetic discharge, with an increase in the right atrial contractility and thus in ventricle filling. The atrium contracts toward the end of the right ventricle diastole. The increase in the force of atrial contractions causes an increase in the pressure within the ventricle and thereby increases the degree of stretching of the myocardium before contraction. Starling's curve states that in the individual muscle fiber, the tension developed on contraction is a function of the initial length before contraction. Applying this relationship to myocardial fibers, a more effective contraction should therefore result from a greater degree of stretching of fibers by increased filling pressure:

↑ atrial contraction → ↑ ventricle filling → ↑ pressure

within ventricle → ↑ diastolic fiber length → and improved

systolic tension

Stimulation of the sympathetic nerve also shifts the ventricular length tension curve to the left, i.e. greater contractility for the same initial length.

Thus, sympathetic stimulation increases the contractility in these three ways:

1. By increasing the atrial contractility and hence the initial stretch of the ventricle's muscle fiber.
2. By acting directly on the ventricle and moving its length tension curve to the left.
3. By increasing the coronary blood flow.

A summary of the neural and humoral regulation of the cardiac function is presented in Figure 22.

TABLE IV

Effects of Stimulation of Parasympathetic and Sympathetic Nerves On the Heart

Parasympathetic

1) Rate of contraction decreases.
2) Shortens refractory period.
3) Decreases atrial excitability.
4) Decreases atrial contractility and hence decreased ventricular filling; does not affect ventricular contractility directly.
5) Prolongation of A.V. conduction time.
6) Decreases in blood flow through the coronary artery.

Sympathetic

1) Rate of contraction increases.
2) Lengthens refractory period.
3) Enhances excitability of atrium and ventricle.
4) Increases atrial contractility and hence increased ventricular filling leading to improved systolic tension.
5) Increases ventricular contractility which is independent of ventricular filling.
6) Shortens ventricular systole and lengthens diastole.
7) Increases in blood flow through the coronary artery.

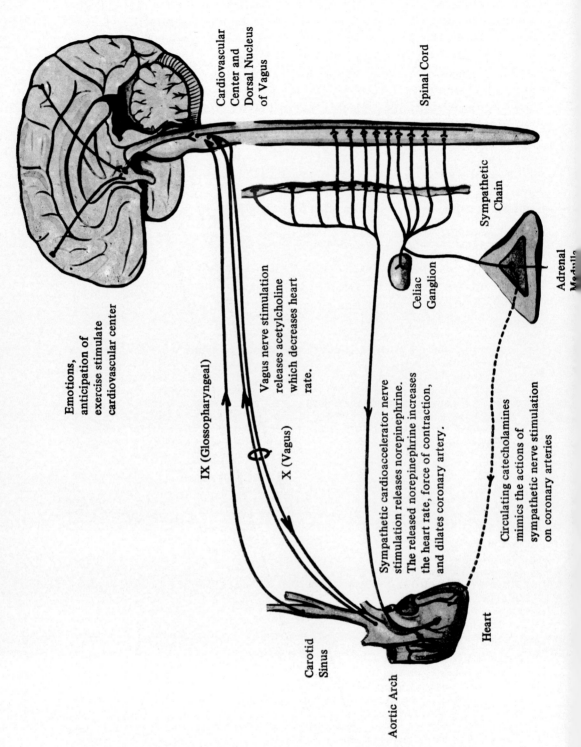

Figure 22. *Schematic Representation of the Neurohumoral Control of the Heart Function*

EFFECT OF CORONARY PERFUSION ON THE FORCE OF CONTRACTION OF THE HEART

The force of contraction of the heart is increased when its oxygen supply is increased by increasing its coronary blood flow and vice versa. Thus the magnitude of force of contraction for a given amount of stretch is also influenced by the metabolic state of the myocardium. The effect of catecholamines in causing coronary dilation is not direct *per se* but is due to increased myocardial metabolites. The circulating catecholamines can greatly increase the work capacity of the heart and thus increase metabolism.

CHAPTER VII

BLOOD VESSELS

STRUCTURE OF VESSELS

THE WHOLE VASCULAR system is distensible and elastic, so that its capacity increases with the increase in blood pressure. Since the heart pumps blood, the pressure which causes the flow of blood through the system must decline as blood flows from the arterial to the venous side. In the arteries the pressure is high, e.g. about 120 mm Hg. in the large arteries of man. The chief function of the large arteries is to serve as elastic conduits, whereas the small arteries and arterioles with their contractile semi-muscular wall leading from the arteries to the capillaries, have in addition, the function of regulating the amount of blood flowing through the capillary area of the organs which they supply. This is done by altering their calibre and hence the resistance to blood flow. These vessels are therefore called "resistance" vessels. In the capillaries the pressure is much lower, 15 to 35 mm Hg. The veins have the function of conducting blood at a low pressure (not usually greater than 5 mm Hg.) from capillaries to heart (Fig. 23). The veins hold any excess of blood which is not immediately taken up by the heart. Accordingly, they are called capacitance vessels.

ARTERIES

The typical artery consists of three coats: the outer or adventitial layer, consisting of collagenous connective tissue and some elastic fibers; the middle layer or media consisting of mainly smooth muscle; and the inner or intimal layer consisting of a smooth endothelial lining containing elastic fibres often formed as an internal elastic membrane. The large arteries are thick-walled and contain an abundance of muscular as well as elastic fibers in their medial walls whereas the medium sized arteries have smooth muscles and less elastic convective tissue in their walls.

The smooth muscle fibers are arranged as layers of the circular muscles in which the individual fibers encircle the lumen. When the circular fibers contract, the lumen becomes smaller resulting in a decrease in the carrying capacity of the arteries. Their relaxation has the opposite effect. The muscles

58

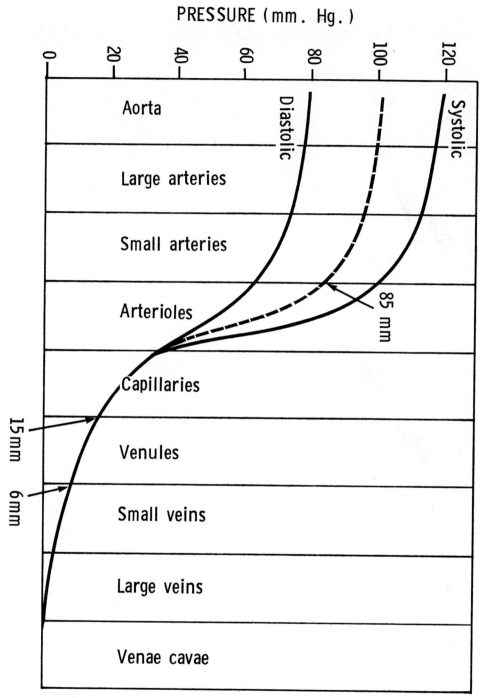

Figure 23. The blood pressure in various parts of the circulation.

are especially abundant in the smaller distributing arteries and arterioles where the bed of the vascular system is large.

Arteries are of two different types, the "distensible" and the "muscular." The calibre of the former depends mainly on the arterial pressure within, whereas calibre of the latter is a balance between the arterial pressure within and the degree of contraction of muscular element.

In the distensible arteries the elastic tissue is most highly developed in those parts of the aorta and of the pulmonary artery nearest the heart, while the muscle fibers are less in evidence. The elastic tissue stretches and the vessels accommodate more blood during the rise of pressure caused by ventricular systole. This elastic buffering action results in a flattening of the pressure peaks and provides a smoother onward flow of blood. The smaller arteries (of the "muscular type") regulate the supply of the blood to various tissues. In arterioles the final arterial element, which is the distensible element, is negligible so that the wall consists of muscle fibers. Numerous arterioles, owing to their small calibre and muscular walls, present the greatest component of resistance to blood flow. Thus, regulation of the blood pressure is accomplished mainly by alterations in the tone of the smooth muscle in the arteriolar walls.

Capillaries

The smallest arterioles branch off into capillaries which contain only a unicellular layer of endothelial cells and is surrounded by a thin basement membrane on the outside; thus it possesses a limited power of contracting and relaxing. Precapillary muscular vessels control the flow of blood into the capillaries and therefore provide the basis for supplying the tissues according to their local metabolic needs (Fig. 24).

The termination of the capillaries on the venous side of the circulation is marked by the reappearance of a slight amount of smooth muscle cells in the media of the venules and a thick layer of collagenous connective tissue in the adventitia.

Veins

The venules unite to form small veins. The same three coats are less distinguishable than in the typical small artery. In the larger veins, the tunica media is not well developed although it does contain some circular smooth muscle. Bundles of longitudinally arranged smooth muscle also appear in the adventitia. The wall of the veins is much thinner in proportion to the lumen. The vein, because of a preponderance of the fibrous tissue elements and the lack of muscular and elastic fibers, tends to collapse unless it is distended by internal fluid pressure.

CONTROL OF THE CALIBRE OF THE BLOOD VESSELS

The calibre of the blood vessel is controlled by several factors. The most

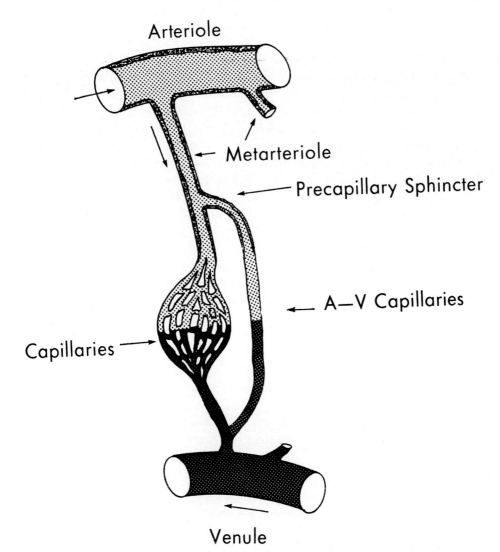

Arteriole

Metarteriole

Precapillary Sphincter

A—V Capillaries

Capillaries

Venule

Figure 24. *Schematic Representation of a Functional Unit of the Capillary Bed.*
The capillary bed is presented as a central channel called arteriolar-venular (a-v) channel of which the capillaries are the side branches. The muscular element is restricted to the first part of the central A-V channels and their branches. These A-V channels remain open under a condition, and consist of four parts: (1) metarterioles, (2) proximal portion, (3) A-V-capillary and (4) venules. A-V capillary and venule have no muscle cell. The venule acquire muscle after it leaves the capillary bed. The true capillary wall consists of a single layer of flattened endothelial cells. Thus there is no resistance to the diffusion of dissolved substances.

important of these factors are (1) myogenic, (2) hormonal, (3) thermal, (4) metabolic and (5) nervous.

Myogenic Responses

In 1902 Bayliss suggested that "the muscular coat of the arteries reacts, like smooth muscle in other situations, to a stretching force by contraction" independent of the nervous system. More recently Folkow *et al.* (1964) have investigated this concept that myogenic tone results from distension of the arterioles by intraluminal pressure in denervated vascular beds and have explained the phenomenon of autoregulation as follows: arterial smooth muscle has intrinsic automaticity; this automaticity is increased when the vascular ring is stretched by increases in intraluminal pressure, and the resultant higher rate of firing leads to stronger contractions until the limit of the muscle's responsiveness is reached. This relationship keeps the perfusion pressure relatively constant at all levels of systemic blood pressure. Local products of metabolism alter the *setting* of the automatic smooth muscle cells in such a way that increased muscular or metabolic activity causes some vasodilatation and results in increased perfusion. A fall of intraluminal pressure would result, according to this hypothesis, in a decrease of vascular tone, and would thus tend to autoregulate flow.

The myogenic activity is particularly pronounced in smooth muscles in the precapillary resistance vessels and sphincters (Fig. 25). It is independent of adrenergic innervation, since a certain degree of tone is maintained in most organs except the skin after complete denervation. This type of constriction is more pronounced where the influence of vasoconstrictor fibers is less apparent. It is manifested even in the absence of blood-born excitatory agents. Certain organs, such as the heart and brain, which are practically devoid of sympathetic vasoconstrictor influences exhibit characteristics of a predominantly local regulation of blood flow which seems to be related to myogenic activity of the vascular smooth muscle. Even the vessels of the splanchnic organs and skeletal muscle show such characteristics.

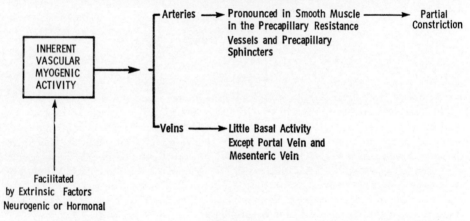

Figure 25

Smooth muscle tone is the consequence of continuous membrane activity. The spontaneously active smooth muscle depends on rhythmically discharged action potentials followed by a mechanical change. Although the rate of discharge may be slow, the result is a fused or partially fused tetanus. Stretch causes a membrane depolarization which results in greater electrical and mechanical activity. Therefore, vascular distension connected with stretch on the smooth muscle cells is a stimulus to contraction and hence to vasoconstriction. Autoregulation of blood flow, which is a tendency for blood flow to remain constant despite changes of perfusion pressure, can at least partly be explained by such a myogenic response.

Metabolic Autoregulation

Several factors are responsible for autoregulation in any one tissue, and the importance of each factor varies with the tissue. The metabolic factor is most prominent in highly metabolizing tissues such as exercising skeletal muscle, heart, and brain and to some extent in the kidney. It is not present in the skin. Due to increase in tissue activity, metabolic substances which are formed act locally on the vascular bed to cause vasodilation. When this occurs, all other influences are rapidly superseded by this most powerful mechanism. Factors which cause decrease in myogenic tone are presented in Figure 26.

The local concentration of metabolites (of a vasodilator nature) varies inversely with the blood flow through the tissue. If flow increases, the metabolites are washed out and flow decreases proportionately.

The metabolites and other substances released during tissue activity or delivered by the blood itself may include oxygen, carbon dioxide, hydrogen

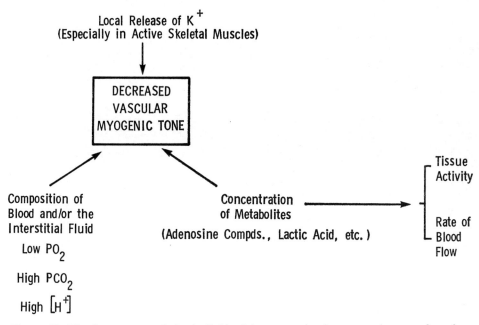

Figure 26. The importance of the individual factors varies from one tissue to the other; and even in the same tissue depending upon time and situation. Adenosine compounds and low PO_2 have powerful effects on the coronaries and [H+] appears to be the main regulator of the cerebral vessels.

ions, adenosine compounds, histamine, bradykinin, prostaglandins, lactic acid, potassium concentration, and plasma osmolarity.

Since all these factors are present to some degree during hyperemia, it is possible that they are collectively responsible for the blood flow patterns seen. For example, during exercise there is an increase in lactic acid and in potassium concentration which could produce vasodilation. Moreover, increased plasma potassium, together with reduced pO_2 acts synergistically to increase blood flow. Plasma osmolarity is also elevated during exercise. It has been proposed that increased plasma osmolarity causes fluid to leave the cells of small arteries and arterioles to reduce their wall thickness and increase their lumen and thus provide for hyperemia. The relative significance and level of interactions between the various metabolites however, probably vary between tissues as well as between species.

These metabolites particularly affect the precapillary vessels, and have relatively little influence on the postcapillary vessels which remain predominantly under the control of sympathetic nervous influence. The characteristic of metabolic autoregulation is presented in Figure 27.

In contrast to resistance vessels the venous capacitance vessels manifest little basal myogenic activity and their tone is determined mainly by the influence of sympathetic vasoconstrictor activity of extrinsic origin. Portal and mesenteric veins, however, contain considerable inherent activity.

The myogenic theory however, does not give a satisfactory general explanation for the mechanism of autoregulation since it cannot explain the pronounced autoregulation of the kidneys and other splanchnic vascular

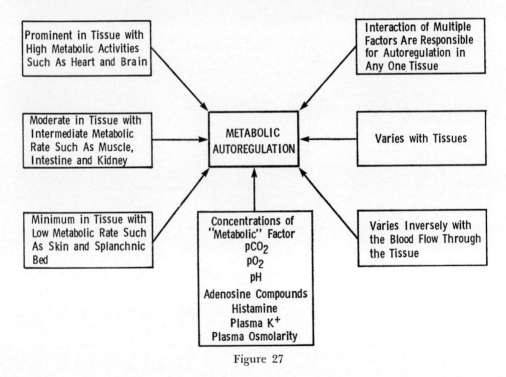

Figure 27

beds. In the kidney it has been suggested that the juxtaglomerular load of sodium plays a role as an autoregulatory factor.

NERVOUS CONTROL OF BLOOD VESSELS

Innervation of the Blood Vessels

All blood vessels except capillaries are supplied with both afferent and efferent nerves (Fig. 28). The afferent nerve fibers concerned in the innervation of the blood vessels are sensory root components of the cerebrospinal nerves. The efferent nerve includes both vasoconstrictor and vasodilator fibers. They are mainly sympathetic. Limited vascular areas are innervated through both sympathetic and parasympathetic nerves.

Sympathetic Fibers

The preganglionic fibers originate mostly from the intermediolateral cell columns of the thoracic and upper lumbar segments of the spinal cord and leave through the ventral roots. Thus, stimulation of the ventral roots of the cervical, lower lumbar and sacral nerves has little or no influence on the blood pressure. The preganglionic fibers run for a short distance through the ventral (or anterior) root and continue into spinal nerves. They exit from the latter nerves by white communicating rami and reach the adjacent segmental sympathetic ganglia, where they synapse or pass through to make a synapse with ganglionic cells higher up or lower down. All of these ganglia are called vertebral or trunk ganglia (Fig. 29). Other preganglionic nerve fibers pass through these vertebral ganglia to end in the collateral ganglia, such as celiac, superior and inferior mesenteric ganglia. As a consequence of this type of arrangement, a widely diffused spread of impulses may result from stimulation of relatively few preganglionic fibers. In fact, as many as eight ganglia can be excited through stimulation of a single anterior root.

The sympathetic ganglion consists of an accumulation of large ganglionic cell bodies, from which arise nonmyelinated class C fibers. The latter may extend up or down the sympathetic trunk for several segments and then may leave through the grey communicating ramus (sympathetic root) to reenter the spinal nerve near the origin of the white communicating ramus. In most instances, however, they exit one or two segments caudal to the point of entry of the preganglionic fibers with which they have synapsed. After leaving the sympathetic trunk, postganglionic fibers may follow various routes to supply the blood vessels.

It is now well known that most of the adrenergic innervation of blood vessels resides in the outer portion of the vessel wall, specifically the adventitia and adventitial-medial junction (Pease, 1962; Falck, 1962; Abraham, 1969; Bevan and Verity, 1967; Maxwell *et al*, 1968; Bevan *et al*, 1969). Most of the sympathetic fibers are vasoconstrictor fibers and they

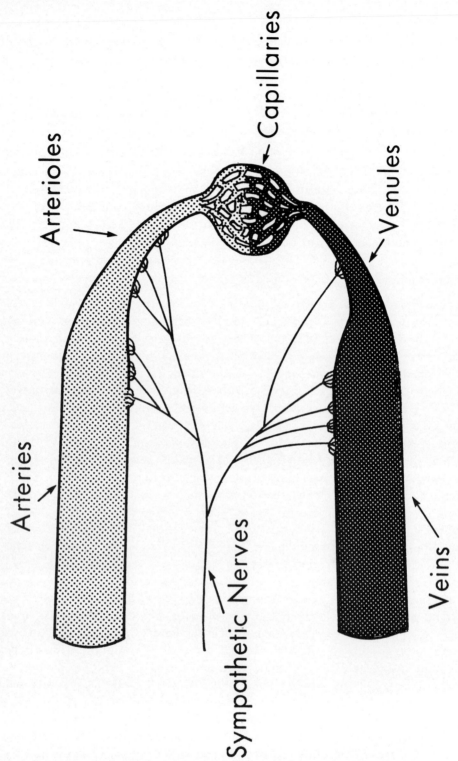

Figure 28. *Schematic representation of the innervation of the blood vessels.*
All arteries and arterioles are innerved with sympathetic nerve fibers. Capillaries have
no sympathetic innervation nor do they respond to sympathetic nerve stimulation. The
venules and veins are also supplied with sympathetic fiber.

release norepinephrine at their nerve endings. Not only is there a cross-sectional localization of norepinephrine in vessels, but also a longitudinal regional concentration.

Large arteries are usually poorly innervated whereas arterioles are densely innervated. The precapillary "sphincters" usually have relatively few adrenergic ramifications.

No sympathetic fibers have been seen to have specific endings in capillaries (Fig. 28), although some axons may run alongside or parallel to these

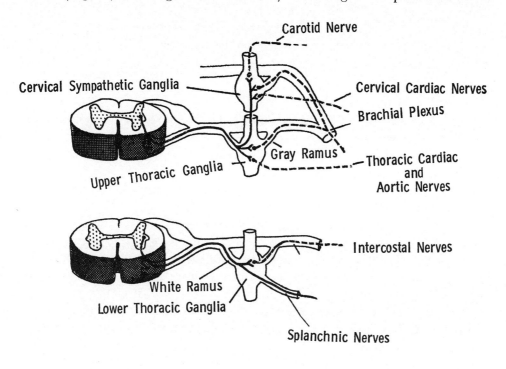

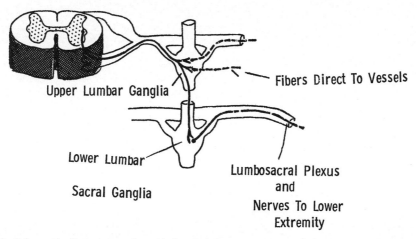

Figure 29. *Schematic Representation of the Origin of Nerves Innervating Blood Vessel.*

vessels for varying distances and single axons are sometimes seen crossing and recrossing the walls of these vessels, often close enough to indent their endothelial lining.

The nerves innervating veins have an arrangement comparable to the arrangement of those which innervate arteries, but the nerve supply of the veins is less abundant than that of the arteries. A very small increase in tone of the veins may considerably alter the venous return to the heart and hence the cardiac output since veins contain about 60 percent of the total blood volume.

The density of adrenergic innervation to different vascular beds is different in different areas. It is sparse in brain whereas it is generous in muscles and skin.

Neurogenic Tone

The vasoconstrictor fibers are tonically active; that is, there is continuous impulse discharge of central nervous origin in the vasoconstrictor nerve to maintain a certain degree of contraction of the smooth muscle in the walls of the blood vessels which is over and above the intrinsic myogenic activity of the effector cells. Inhibition of the tonic discharge of vasoconstrictor impulses causes vasodilation.

The physiological discharge rate in sympathetic fibers is low, about 1 to 3 impulses/sec. The rate increases, however, to about 10 impulses/sec during intense asphyxia. Sympathetic vasoconstrictor fibers are generally believed to play a very important role in regulating peripheral blood flow, particularly in the distal portions of the limbs.

There are, however, great regional differences of the sympathetic vasoconstrictor fiber influences. Sympathetic tone is prominent on the capacitance side of the circulation (vein). It is very pronounced for cutaneous circulation. There is moderate sympathetic vasoconstrictor influence in skeletal muscle whereas sympathetic tone has little influence on the vascular beds in such vital tissues as the brain and myocardium.

VASODILATOR FIBERS

Vasodilatation can be brought about by a release of sympathetic vasoconstrictor tone, or locally induced by some mechanism of autoregulation. Apart from these mechanisms active vasodilatation can be brought about by activation of specific vasodilator fibers which supply blood vessels in some parts of the body (Fig. 30).

There are three types of vasodilator fibres: parasympathetic, sympathetic (Fig. 30), and dorsal root (or antidromic) fibers (Fig. 32).

Parasympathetic Vasodilator Fibers

Such fibers run in certain nerves of the cranial parasympathetic outflow, and also in the sacral outflow (Fig. 31). They innervate blood vessels in the

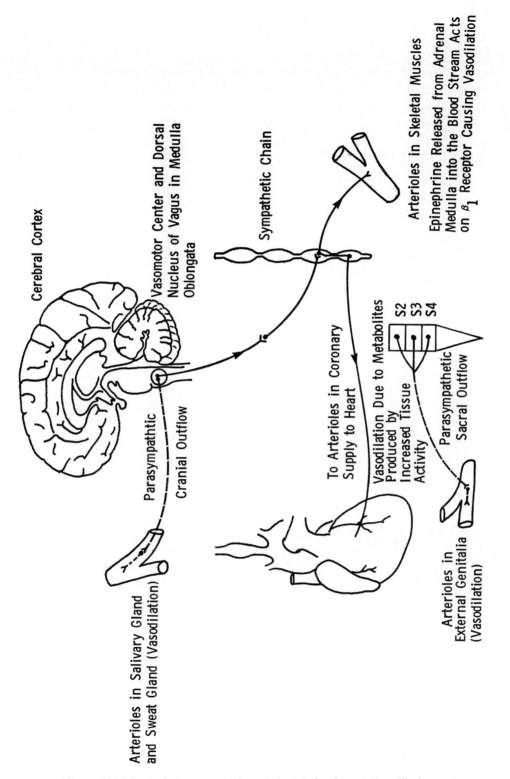

Figure 30. *Schematic Representation of the Mechanism of Vasodilation.*

salivary glands, the pial vessels in the brain, the external genital organs, the lungs and in certain abdominal viscera. Thus, if the chorda tympani nerve is cut, no change is evident in the blood vessels of the submaximallary gland. On the other hand, if its peripheral end is stimulated, there is a secretion of saliva and the blood vessels in the gland dilate. Engorgement of genital erectile tissue occurs when the parasympathetic component of the second and third sacral roots are excited.

Sympathetic Vasodilator Fibers

Some fibers belonging to the sympathetic system are vasodilator in function. When the sympathetic chain in the lumbar region of cats or dogs

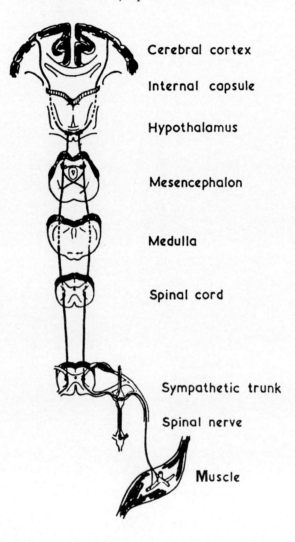

Cerebral cortex

Internal capsule

Hypothalamus

Mesencephalon

Medulla

Spinal cord

Sympathetic trunk

Spinal nerve

Muscle

Figure 31. Schematic diagram of the central and peripheral course of the sympathetic vasodilator pathways. (From Lindgren, P.: The Mesencephalon and the Vasomotor System (An Experimental Study on the Central Control of Peripheral Blood Flow in the Cat), Acta Physiol. Scandinav. 35 (Supp. 121) :175, Fig. 58, 1955).

The cholinergic sympathetic fibers originate in the cerebral cortex relays in the hypothalmus. The efferent fibers from both sides of the hypothalmus are interconnected. From hypothalamus they relay in the mesencephalon and pass through the ventral aspect of the medulla to the preganglionic neurons in the lateral horn cells of the spinal cord. In their passage through the medulla they make no connection with either the pressor or depressor areas and do not participate in reflexes initiated from the carotid sinuses or aortic arch. This pathway is responsible for causing initial rapid dilation of the arterioles in muscle during exercise. Emotional stimuli such as fear and apprehension increase muscle blood flow probably by stimulating this system.

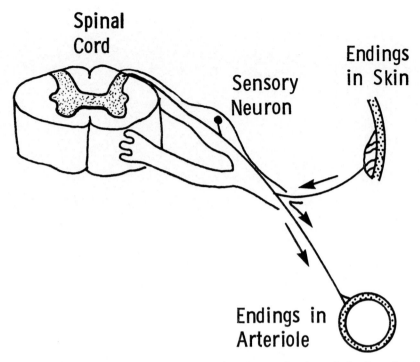

Spinal Cord

Sensory Neuron

Endings in Skin

Endings in Arteriole

Figure 32. *Schematic Representation of Antidromic Conduction of the Impulse to the Periphery.* Impulses generated from the sensory endings in the skin, not only travel to the spinal cord but also by the axon reflex pathway to the arterioles of the skin causes vasodilation and flare.

is stimulated, there is initial dilation followed by constriction in the vascular beds within skeletal muscle. After α-adrenergic receptor blockage, only vasodilation occurs. The vasodilator response is restricted only to skeletal muscle and is potentiated by eserine and antagonized by atropine. Because a substance like acetylcholine is found in the effluent perfusate from such muscles, the fibers concerned are therefore considered to be cholinergic, though sympathetic (Fig. 34). This vascular regulatory system originates in the motor cortex and impulses descend from there to the hypothalamus, pass through the medullary centers without making any connections in the medulla and leave the spinal cord with the sympathetic nerves (Fig. 31). Upon stimulation of these fibers, muscle blood flow becomes five or six times greater.

When the motor cortex initiates muscle activity it simultaneously excites the vasodilator fibers to the active muscles, and vasodilatation occurs immediately, several seconds before the local regulatory vasodilatation can take place. It seems that this vasodilator system has the important function of initiating extra blood flow through the muscles at the onset of muscular activity. It does not exert any tonic influence over the blood vessels nor is it called into play in blood pressure homeostatic mechanisms. Thus, the

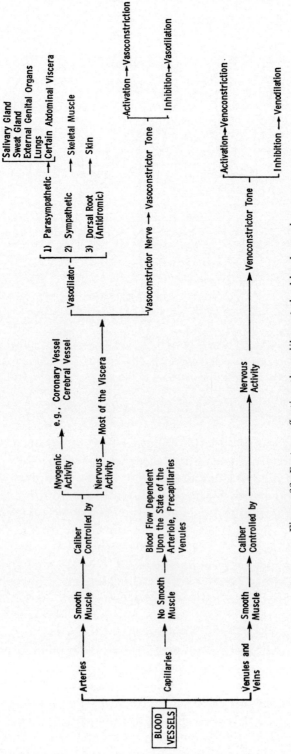

Figure 33. *Factors affecting the caliber of the blood vessels.*

Relative importance of various factors is difficult to determine. Furthermore, reactivity of the smooth musculature to various factors varies greatly in different parts of the vascular system.

sympathetic vasodilator system is in some way involved in the integrative control of muscle blood flow as part of an emotional response pattern concerned with fear, anger, etc., mediated by the hypothalamus.

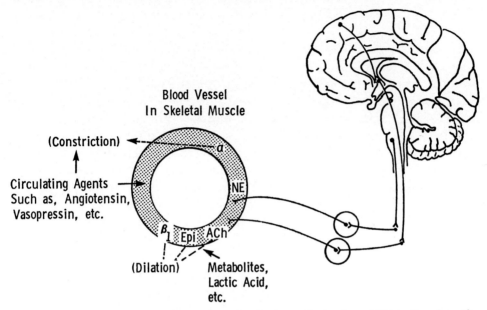

Figure 34. *Schematic Representation of the Various Mechanisms Which Regulate the Blood Flow in Skeletal Muscle.*

ANTIDROMIC VASODILATOR FIBERS

Stimulation of the peripheral ends of several dorsal roots (afferent fibers) causes dilation of the vessels in the area of skin. It appears that sensory nerve fibers in the skin may have collateral fibers distributed to adjacent blood vessels. On stimulation of the sensory endings impulses travel not only to the spinal cord but also to the dilator termination in the blood vessel (Fig. 32), producing vasodilation and flare. Since the impulses on artificial stimulation pass in a direction opposite to that taken by the normal impulses, Bayliss designated them antidromic impulses. The transmitter that they release is yet unidentified but it causes vasodilation and increases capillary permeability.

Control of blood vessels is summarized in Figure 33.

CIRCULATION IN THE SKIN

Circulation to the skin subserves mainly three purposes:

1. nutrition of the skin tissues.

2. a reservoir when there is need for shunting blood to inactive structures and thereby contributing greatly to the control of blood pressure.

3. conduction of the heat from the internal structures to periphery for dissipation even to the point of sacrificing local metabolic needs to maintain body temperature at a normal level.

Cutaneous circulatory apparatus of the skin consists of two major types of vessels: (1) the usual nutritive arteries, capillaries and veins and (2) special vascular structures concerned with heating the skin, consisting principally of (a) an extensive subcutaneous venous plexus, which holds large quantities of blood, and (b) in some skin areas, arteriovenous anastomoses which are highly specialized types of vessels that enable blood to bypass the capillary bed by entering directly into venous channels from small-sized arteries and arterioles. Each unit consists of (1) an arterial or arteriolar portion that arises from a vessel up to 100μ in diameter, (2) an intermediate controlling segment (the capillary bed) and 3) a generally funnel-shaped venous portion that terminates in a vein 50 to 150μ in diameter. The arterio-venous shunt has a very small lumen whereas its wall is two or three times as thick as an arteriole of similar size. They are innervated entirely via sympathetic vasoconstrictor fibers controlled by the hypothalamic heat regulating center. This center modulates the skin blood flow in accord with the body's need.

Flushing of the skin from embarrassment or emotional stimuli also represents vascular changes mediated through higher central nervous centers.

When skin is warmed locally, a vasodilation occurs. This is not due to direct action of the heat on the blood vessels, but due to the release of constrictor tone. Application of excessive cold to the skin may produce a transient vasodilation which may also be independent of the nerve supply.

Having no myogenic tone, the basal tone of these vascular channels is due only to the sympathetic vasoconstrictor fibers. Cutaneous vessels therefore dilate maximally when the sympathetic constrictor influence on them is eliminated by denervation, or by α-receptor blockade, the full range of cutaneous flow can be achieved. There are no sympathetic or parasympathetic vasodilator fibers directly affecting the cutaneous vessels. Injection of acetylcholine induces a slight dilation of these vessels which suggests the presence of noninnervated cholinergic receptors.

Under basal conditions, the overall resistance to blood flow is only moderate in the skin, as a whole, being much greater than that in the cerebral or renal vessels, but it is much less than the resistance imposed by the vessels of the skeletal muscles.

CIRCULATION IN THE SKELETAL MUSCLE

Blood vessels supplying skeletal muscle possess an intrinsic tone which is independent of any innervation. However, the blood vessels in muscle are also supplied with both sympathetic vasoconstrictor fibers and sympathetic vasodilator fibers.

The sympathetic vasoconstrictor fibers maintain the blood vessels in a state of tonic constriction over and above the intrinsic tone. When stimulated maximally, they decrease the blood flow through the skeletal muscle to about $\frac{1}{4}$ of the normal. When this sympathetic vasoconstrictor mechanism is eliminated by sympathetic denervation or after α-receptors block-

TABLE V

Differences in the Skin and Muscle Circulation

Some vascular mechanisms controlling blood vessel caliber appear to have different effects upon the blood vessels in the skin and those in the muscle.

	SKIN	MUSCLE
TONE		
Myogenic	+	+ + +
Vasoconstrictor	+ + +	+
RECEPTORS		
Alpha	+ + +	+
Beta	—	+ + +
MICROCIRCULATION		
Ateriovenous Shunts	+ +	—

ade, the blood vessels still maintain a substantial tone. In addition to the α-receptors there are β-adrenergic receptors (β_1) which are activated by circulating epinephrine resulting in vasodilation.

The vasodilator fibers are cholinergic fibers since they release acetylcholine at their nerve endings. On stimulation they cause maximal dilation. The response can be antagonized by atropine and enhanced by eserine (Fig. 34).

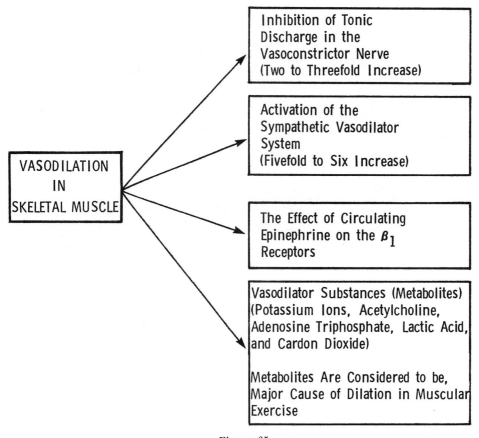

Figure 35

In exercise there is great increase in skeletal muscle blood flow. Maximal exercise may increase the muscle blood flow from a resting value of 2 to 5 ml/100g/min to an average value of 50 to 75 ml/100g/min. However, the degree of vasodilation is nearly the same in normal and denervated limbs and is therefore independent of nervous influence.

The factors which may cause vasodilation in the skeletal muscles are summarized in Figure 35. The most important factor controlling the blood flow in the skeletal muscle is local regulation. Metabolites such as adenosine compounds, potassium ions, lactic acid, carbon dioxide and some unidentified substances released during muscle contraction play an important role in muscle blood flow during muscle activity. They act directly on arterioles to cause vasodilatation. The relative importance of each in increasing muscle blood flow during muscle activity is not known.

The differences in the cutaneous (skin) and skeletal muscular circulations are presented in Table V.

CHAPTER VIII

REGULATION OF BLOOD PRESSURE

MANY FACTORS ARE involved in the complex homeostatic mechanism which maintains normal blood pressure. These include: (1) the baroreceptors in the carotid sinus and aortic arch; (2) the cardioregulatory centers; (3) the chromaffin system; (4) the adrenal-pituitary axis; and (5) the response of the arterioles to constricting stimuli. All these factors integrate to maintain blood pressure levels.

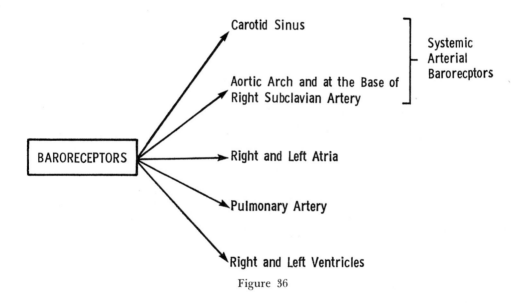

Figure 36

BARORECEPTOR FUNCTION

In several portions of the vascular tree there are present sensory areas called baroreceptors which are sensitive to stretch (Fig. 36). The baroreceptor system involving the carotid sinus reflex is most important for opposing rapid changes in arterial pressure, through sudden changes in posture, alterations in blood volume, acute deterioration of myocardial function, or other acute circulatory stresses that might raise or lower the blood pressure.

From the arch of the aorta three large arteries originate: The innominate, the left common carotid and the left subclavian artery. The innominate artery gives rise to the right common carotid. The common carotid arteries divide into the internal carotid and the external carotid arteries. Upon the internal carotid artery and near its origin from the common carotid are found sensory areas known as the carotid sinuses. Similar sensory areas are found in the arch of the aorta.

The baroreceptors are located in the walls of the blood vessels of the aortic and carotid sinus areas and respond to the pressure in the lumen of the vessels (Fig. 37). They are connected by means of the aortic and carotid sinus nerve to the autonomic center in the medullary area.

These receptors are effectively quiescent when blood pressures are below 60 mm Hg; with the increase in transmural pressure above 60 mm Hg, the frequency increases progressively. The change in frequency of impulses per millimeter mercury pressure change is maximum at about normal blood pressure and reaches a plateau at about 160 mm Hg, i.e. further increases in pressure do not cause any significant increase in the rate of receptor discharge. Thus, when the blood pressure falls below about 60 mm Hg or increases above about 160 mm Hg, this reflex system elicits little further compensatory response.

The efferent pathway of this self-adjustment of arterial pressure is as follows:

1. Vagus and cardiac sympathetic nerve, adjusting heart rate, myocardial contractility and cardiac output.
2. Sympathetic vasomotor nerves, adjusting the peripheral vasomotor tone of the resistance and capacity vessels.
3. Sympathetic nerves, regulating the epinephrine and norepinephrine secretion of the adrenal medullary glands. These hormones may also affect the heart rate, myocardial contractility, cardiac output and peripheral vascular resistance and capacity.

When the blood pressure increases, the baroreceptors are stimulated. Nerve impulses initiated ascend by way of aortic and carotid sinus nerves to reach the cardiac and vasomotor centers. The baroreceptors' activity inhibits the vasomotor center. Efferent impulses over the vagus nerves inhibit the heart, thereby slowing its force and rate of contraction. Other impulses descend to the spinal cord and cause reduction in vasoconstrictor tone, resulting in dilation of the blood vessels (Fig. 37). Their resistance

Figure 37. Schematic representation of the mechanism that tends to maintain the arterial blood pressure. Under normal conditions baro-receptors' (aortic arch and carotid sinus) activity partially inhibits the vasomotor center maintaining a normal arteriolar tone (A). Higher blood pressure stimulates the aortic and carotid baroreceptors. This leads to increased inhibitory impulses to the vasomotor center resulting in a reduction of vasomotor tone. This results in vasodilation of the arteries which then restores normal blood pressure (B). On the other hand when blood pressure falls there is a decrease in baroreceptor activity resulting in a reduction in the inhibition of the vasomotor center. This leads to more impulses per sec over vasomotor nerves. As a result vasoconstriction occurs and the blood pressure is restored to normal level.

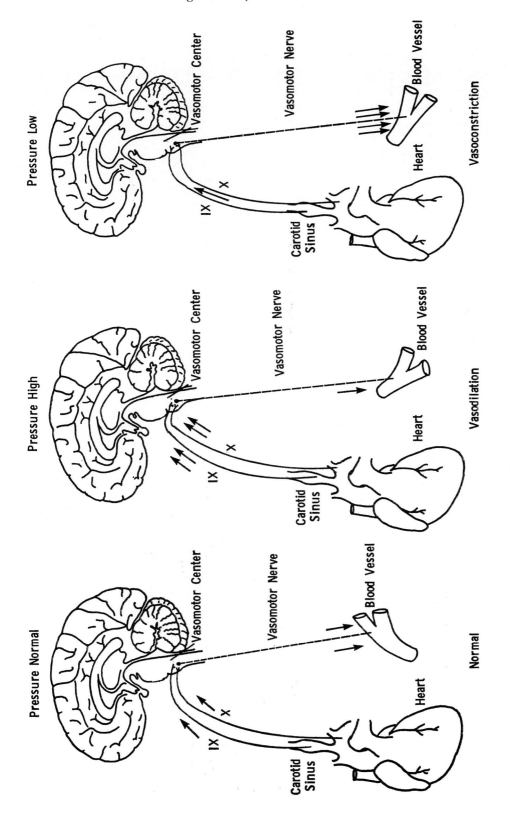

to the blood decreases and blood pressure thus falls. With the decrease in pressure, stimulation of the carotid and aortic receptors is reduced. Therefore, fewer impulses reach the cardioregulatory center and there is less inhibition of the vasomotor center (Fig. 37). The reflex arc produces effects in approximately three to four seconds.

This arterial baroreceptor reflex is also important in antagonizing a fall in blood pressure. When blood pressure declines, fewer afferent impulses

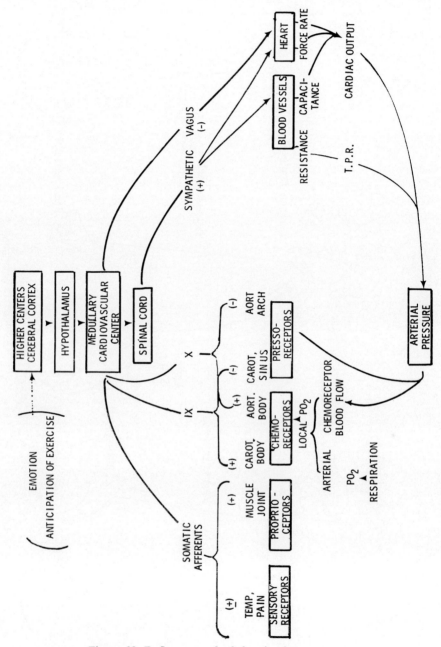

Figure 38. Reflex control of the circulatory system.

THE SYMPATHETIC CONTROL OF THE CIRCULATORY SYSTEM IS COMPLEX AND INVOLVES LEVELS OF INTEGRATION IN THE CENTRAL NERVOUS SYSTEM.

LEVEL	INTEGRATION
1) Spinal cord	Coarse control, e.g., segmental reflexes
2) Medulla oblongata	Main control of blood pressure and cardiac function
3) Hypothalamus	Fine control of regional flows, and integration of circulatory control with respiratory and thermoregulatory systems
4) Cortex	Integration of circulatory control with somatic motor system, e.g., increased muscle bloodflow with exercise

Figure 39

Figure 40. Schematic representation of the factors affecting the vasomotor center.

Because of continuous central sympathetic nervous impulse discharge, the blood vessels are normally held in a state of tonic constriction. Changes in the rate of impulse discharge alter the vascular tone to meet physiological demands. The sympathetic vasoconstrictor nerves are under the control of the vasomotor centre which is located in the floor of the fourth ventricle at the apex of the calamus scriptoris and in close anatomical and functional association with the cardiac and respiratory centres. The vasomotor centre is sensitive to the pCO_2 and pO_2 of the blood passing through it and it is influenced by nerve impulses originating from other parts of the central nervous system (the other medullary centers, the hypothalamus and the higher reaches of the brain, and from the periphery). For physiological control of the blood vessels, the most important are the pressor receptors of the carotid sinus and the aortic arch. The corresponding chemoreceptors (in the carotid and aortic bodies) are also linked with the vasomotor centre but they are more important in respiratory than in vasomotor control.

from the pressoreceptors go to the cardiovascular centers. Therefore, vagus tone is decreased, and consequently there is less inhibition of the sympathetic division. As a result, cardiac action and vasoconstriction increases. For example, when blood pressure tends to fall following hemorrhage, it leads to increased sympathetic activity. Reflex control of the circulatory system is schematically presented in Figure 38.

Higher hypothalamic centers can temporarily suspend baroreceptor con-

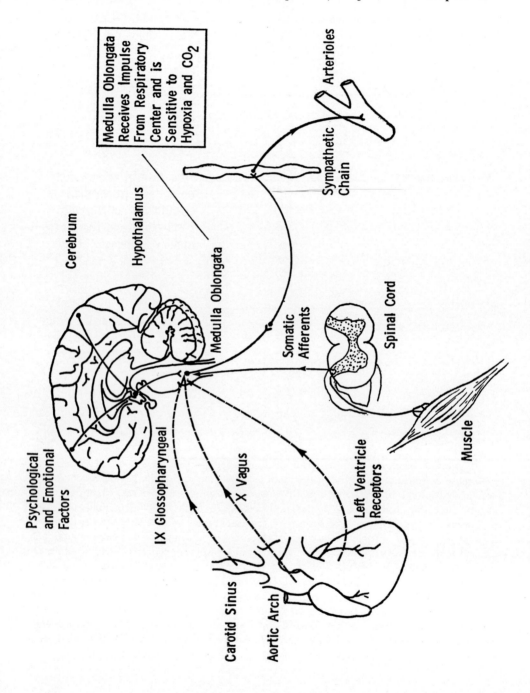

trol of vasomotor output (Fig. 40). This can be seen in instances of fear, rage, and anger where baroreceptor inhibition of sympathetic discharge is partially or completely removed. These mechanisms serve a useful purpose in daily life and are part of Cannon's emergency reflex. There is no convincing evidence that these higher centers have more than a temporary modifying effect on the basic medullary blood pressure control system.

The sympathetic control of the circulatory system involves several levels of integration in the central nervous system (Fig. 39). They include: (1) the cerebral cortex, (2) the hypothalamus, (3) the cardiovascular system in the medulla oblongata, and (4) the spinal cord. The function of these centers is modified by (1) emotional stimuli; (2) stimuli coming from various parts of the body over visceral and somatic afferents; (3) variation in CO_2 and O_2 tension; (4) and changes in pH.

The main integration of sympathetic afferent impulses and the origination of efferent impulses for the homeostatic control of Cardiovascular system takes place in the medulla oblongata (Figs. 40, 41).

The cardiovascular control centers in the medulla oblongata receive impulses from higher parts of the brain, giving rise to changes in heart rate and blood pressure associated with emotional conditions.

The hypothalamus plays an important role in the control of the vasoconstrictor system. It has no tonic activity. The postero-lateral portion of the hypothalamus exerts powerful excitation whereas the anterior portion can either cause excitation or inhibition depending upon the location of stimulation. Redistribution of blood flow and characteristic pattern of cardiovascular response are integrated at this level. The cardiovascular adjustment to emotions such as rage are mediated here.

Reflexes may also be integrated at the level of the spinal cord, and it is evident that the cord is not completely subservient to higher levels of the central nervous system.

MEDULLARY CONTROL

The main cardiovascular control centers are located in the medulla. Stimulation of some areas in the medulla oblongata causes an excitatory response, whereas stimulation of other areas produces an inhibitory response. These areas are not strictly localized, but represent rather a diffuse network of interconnected groups of neurons in the reticular formation. The areas which control the heart are closely associated with those which control the vascular system. For the sake of convenience, the medullary cardiovascular center is divided into three parts:

1. Vasomotor center
2. Cardio-inhibitory center
3. Cardio-excitatory center

The medullary centers receive impulses from all parts of the body, i.e. from peripheral sensors and from higher brain centers. These medullary centers integrate all the afferent impulses and they give rise to the efferent

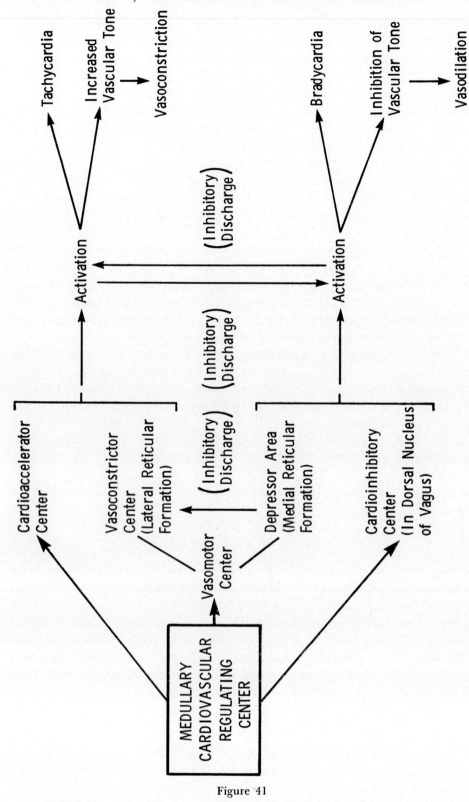

Figure 41

impulses for cardiovascular homeostasis (Fig. 41). They regulate the blood pressure, the cardiac output and the flow distribution even when the centers are disconnected from higher nervous structures.

Vasomotor Center

The vasomotor center is located bilaterally in the reticular formation and extends from the lower part of the pons to the obex. Its existence was noticed by Carl Ludwig in 1870. When descending serial transections of the brain stem are made, blood pressure remains relatively constant until a section is made at the level of the obex. At this point blood pressure drops. Results obtained from electrical stimulation of various parts of the medulla indicate that the vasomotor center may be divided into two functional areas: a pressor area in the lateral reticular formation (Alexander, 1946) and a depressor area in the medial reticular formation. The stimulation of a pressor area causes a rise in blood pressure due to excitation of vasoconstrictor neurons. It is therefore called the vasoconstrictor center. The vasoconstrictor neurons have inherent activity independent of the afferent stimuli. There is a continuous discharge from the area in essentially all vasoconstrictor nerve fibers of the body. The discharge is at a slow rate of about one half to two impulses per second. This impulse discharge is responsible for the neurogenic component of basal vasoconstrictor tone and maintains a partial state of contraction of all blood vessels to half of their normal diameter. The stimulation of the vasodepressor area causes vasodilation. This vasodilation is due to an inhibition of vasoconstrictor tone and not to an activation of specific vasodilator fibers. These two areas act as a functional unit.

The Cardio-Inhibitory Center

The cardio-inhibitory center is in the dorsal nucleus of the vagus and gives rise to the efferent fibers of the vagus. Direct stimulation causes slowing or stoppage of the heart. The vagal cardio-inhibitory *center* is tonically active mainly due to the input from the baroreceptors; it has little or no inherent activity. When carotid sinus and aortic nerves are sectioned, vagal tone is virtually abolished.

Functionally, the cardio-inhibitory center is closely associated with the vasodepressor area of the vasomotor center so that excitation of both simultaneously elicits slowing of the heart and peripheral vasodilation. The vasodilation is due to an inhibition of sympathetic vasoconstrictor tone. These effects are mediated therefore by both the parasympathetic (to the heart only) and sympathetic (to the heart and blood vessels) systems.

The Cardio-Excitatory Center

The cardio-excitatory center is closely associated with the vasoconstrictor center functionally. These two centers, i.e. the vasoconstrictor center and

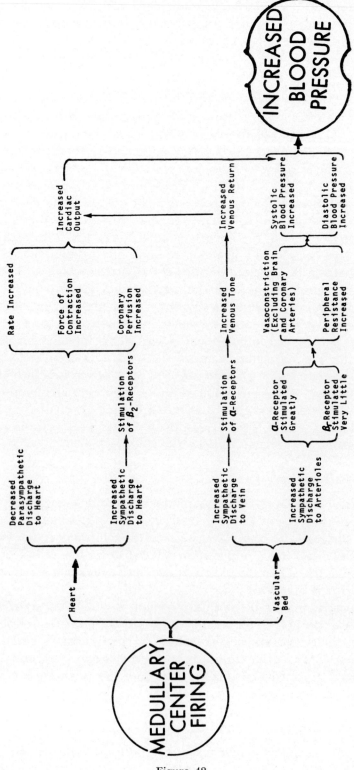

Figure 42

the cardioaccelerator center, send outflow down the spinal cord which is distributed to the nodal tissue in the heart, heart muscle and peripheral vessels by way of the sympathetic nervous system.

Activation of these cells leads to tachycardia and peripheral vasoconstriction.

There appears to be an intimate neural relationship between the cardioinhibitory center and the cardioaccelerator center, both exerting an inhibitory influence on each other.

The medullary cardiovascular regulating center is schematically presented in Figure 41.

Respiratory Center

The cardiovascular system is influenced greatly by the respiratory system since the medullary respiratory neurons are intermingled with those of pressor areas of the cardiovascular system. This is seen by fluctuations in arterial blood pressure (Traube-Hering waves) and a complex pattern of heart rate changes (sinus arrhythmia) related to respiratory activity. Arterial pressoreceptor discharge inhibits not only cardiac and vascular activity but also respiration.

EFFECT OF ALTERATION IN THE DISCHARGE OF THE MEDULLARY NEURONS

Most emotional reactions of the nervous system can temporarily affect the cardiovascular system. They exert their effects via the medullary centers, i.e. impulses coming from the various areas of the brain, particularly from the hypothalamus, descend to the medulla and through synaptic connections alter the discharge of the primary medullary neurons. For example, increasing the levels of excitement as usually occurs in sudden anger increases the rate of medullary discharge resulting in a rise in blood pressure (Fig. 42).

A particularly interesting circulatory reaction occurs in a person who faints because of an intense emotional experience. In these circumstances, there is activation of sympathetic vasodilator system so that the blood flow through the muscle increases several times. Concomitantly, impulses from higher centers act upon the vasomotor center in the medulla oblongata to inhibit sympathetic activity and enhance parasympathetic activity. The heart rate falls steeply due to vagal inhibition; the peripheral resistance drops. Due to extensive vasodilation, blood pressure falls. The blood supply to the brain is inadequate and there is a loss of consciousness (Fig. 43).

⟶

Figure 43. Role of Autonomic Nervous System in Fainting in Response to Strong Emotional Stimulus.

Strong emotional stimulus exerts an inhibitory effect upon the medullary cardiovascular centers resulting in a decreased sympathetic discharge and enhanced parasympathetic activity.

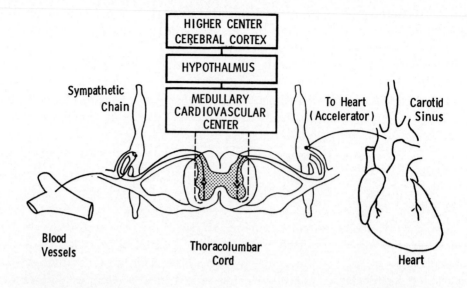

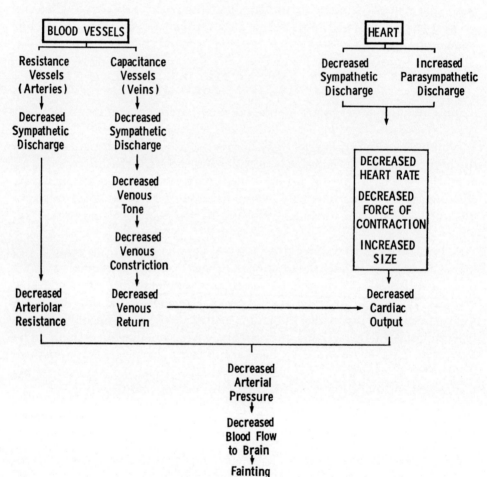

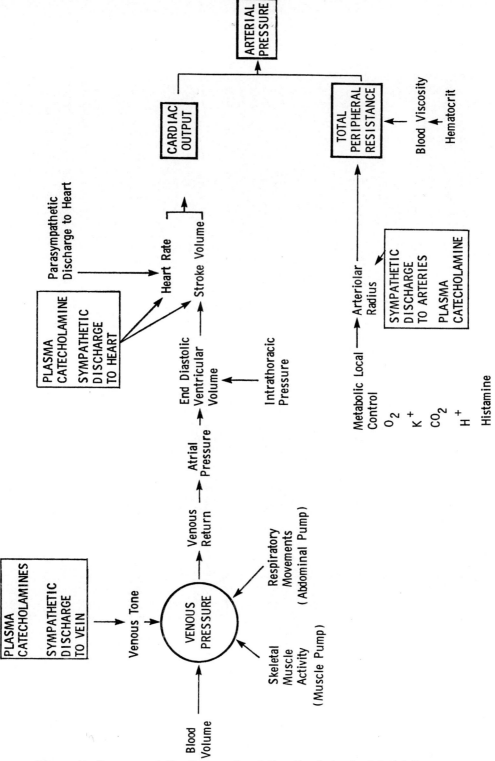

Figure 44. *Summary of the Factors Regulating the Systemic Arterial Pressure.*
The blood pressure is maintained by an integration of (1) cardiac output, (2) peripheral resistance, (3) elasticity of the main arteries, (4) viscosity of the blood and (5) blood volume.

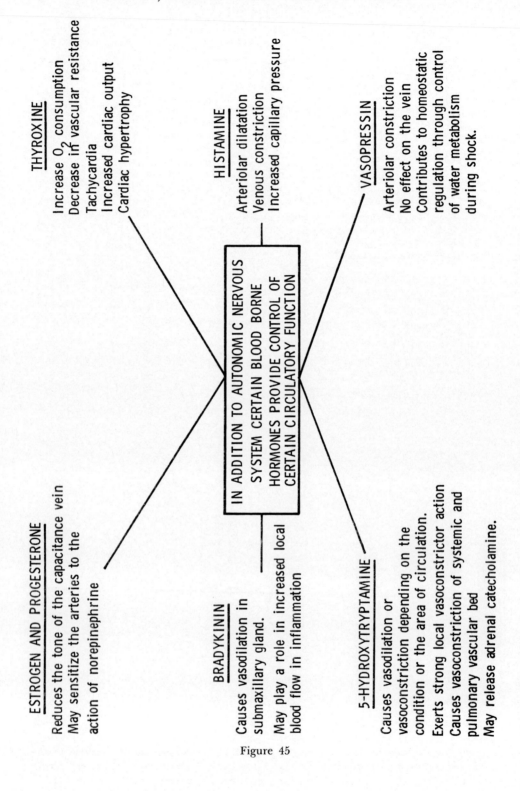

THYROXINE

Increase O$_2$ consumption
Decrease in vascular resistance
Tachycardia
Increased cardiac output
Cardiac hypertrophy

HISTAMINE

Arteriolar dilatation
Venous constriction
Increased capillary pressure

VASOPRESSIN

Arteriolar constriction
No effect on the vein
Contributes to homeostatic
regulation through control
of water metabolism
during shock.

ESTROGEN AND PROGESTERONE

Reduces the tone of the capacitance vein
May sensitize the arteries to the
action of norepinephrine

BRADYKININ

Causes vasodilation in
submaxillary gland.
May play a role in increased local
blood flow in inflammation

5-HYDROXYTRYPTAMINE

Causes vasodilation or
vasoconstriction depending on the
condition or the area of circulation.
Exerts strong local vasoconstrictor action
Causes vasoconstriction of systemic and
pulmonary vascular bed
May release adrenal catecholamine.

IN ADDITION TO AUTONOMIC NERVOUS
SYSTEM CERTAIN BLOOD BORNE
HORMONES PROVIDE CONTROL OF
CERTAIN CIRCULATORY FUNCTION

Figure 45

Ordinarily, cerebral blood flow is independent of arterial blood pressure except at very low pressure. To maintain cerebral perfusion, only a mean arterial pressure of approximately 40–50 mm Hg is necessary, it is therefore apparent that only a reduction of blood pressure to extremely low levels will induce fainting.

Summary of the neural control of the blood pressure is presented in Figure 44.

HORMONAL CONTROL OF THE CARDIOVASCULAR SYSTEM

Although the autonomic nervous system provides the dominant regulatory mechanism for the circulatory system, certain blood-born hormones also may affect the control of certain circulatory functions. Certain of these hormones exert their action by interacting with the autonomic nervous system directly or indirectly whereas others act independently. The actions of the most important of these hormones are presented in Figure 45.

THE CIRCULATORY CHANGES DURING MUSCULAR EXERCISE

Several factors are normally involved simultaneously in the adaptation of the cardiovascular system to the necessities of the body. For example, during muscular exercise there are changes in: (a) release of catecholamines, (b) cardiac output, (c) blood flow in the tissue, (d) peripheral resistance and blood pressure and (e) venous pressure.

Release of Catecholamines

Anticipation of exercise stimulates the cardioregulatory centers which increase the rate of sympathetic discharge, resulting in a release of catecholamines from the sympathetic nerve endings as well as from the suprarenal medulla. The release of catecholamines is increased further during exercise.

Catecholamines released locally at the sinoatrial node stimulate the heart rate. Catecholamines in the blood enter the heart via the coronary arteries and cause dilation, thus improving the O_2 delivery to the myocardium. This improves the cardiac work capacity and accelerates the myocardial oxidative metabolism. The increased release of local metabolites causes further coronary dilation.

Cardiac Output

The cardiac output at rest is of the order of 6 to 8 liters/min for the upright individual and increases linearly with increasing O_2 uptake, to reach levels as high as 25 to 30 liters/min in healthy young athletes during heavy exhausting exercise. For those people who are healthy but who are not as young or as fit, maximum cardiac output would commonly fall in the range of 20 to 25 liters/min. The increase in cardiac output during exercise is due partly to an increase in stroke volume (which approximately doubles), while the remaining contribution is due to the increase in heart rate.

Redistribution of Blood

In order to increase the blood flow to active tissue, the entire circulatory system is coordinated. The increased blood flow to the active muscles is accomplished not only by an increase in total cardiac output but also by redistribution of regional blood flows.

During exercise, there is an increase in sympathetic discharge, which causes vasoconstriction in the vascular beds of the liver, the splanchnic area, the kidney and at the start of exercise, in the skin. The blood flow to these areas is consequently reduced, thereby allowing a greater proportion of the cardiac output to be available for the exercising muscles. The blood flow to non-exercising skeletal muscles is similarly diminished. As the exercise continues, the need to eliminate heat from the body requires an increase in the blood flow to the skin.

The blood flow to the exercising skeletal muscles is increased because of vasodilation due mainly to increased release of metabolites, although the action of circulating epinephrine on beta-receptors also plays a part. The cerebral circulation is maintained during moderate activity, but blood flow is decreased during maximal exercise in response to a fall in carbon dioxide tension that accompanies hyperventilation. The circulation in the skin varies with the intensity and duration of exercise. It is decreased at first because of sympathetic discharges. There is dilation of blood vessels and the flow increases in order to eliminate the excessive heat produced by the increase in metabolic rate. If exercise is continued, however, the effect of catecholamines override, and there is vasoconstriction, despite the need for heat dissipation.

Peripheral Resistance and Blood Pressure

In rhythmic exercise, the total peripheral resistance is decreased by an amount proportional to the degree of exercise undertaken. The increase in blood pressure is entirely due to increase in cardiac output.

Venous Return

In response to the increase in sympathetic discharge, venoconstriction occurs. This decreases the capacity of the venous bed and aids the venous return to the heart. The phasic contraction of the skeletal muscles during exercise and respiratory movement during exercise act as a pump and thus aid in increasing the venous return. The increase in venous return is responsible for increased cardiac output.

(↑venous return - - - ↑stroke volume - - - ↑cardiac output)

Thus, during exercise there is (a) an increase in release of catecholamine,

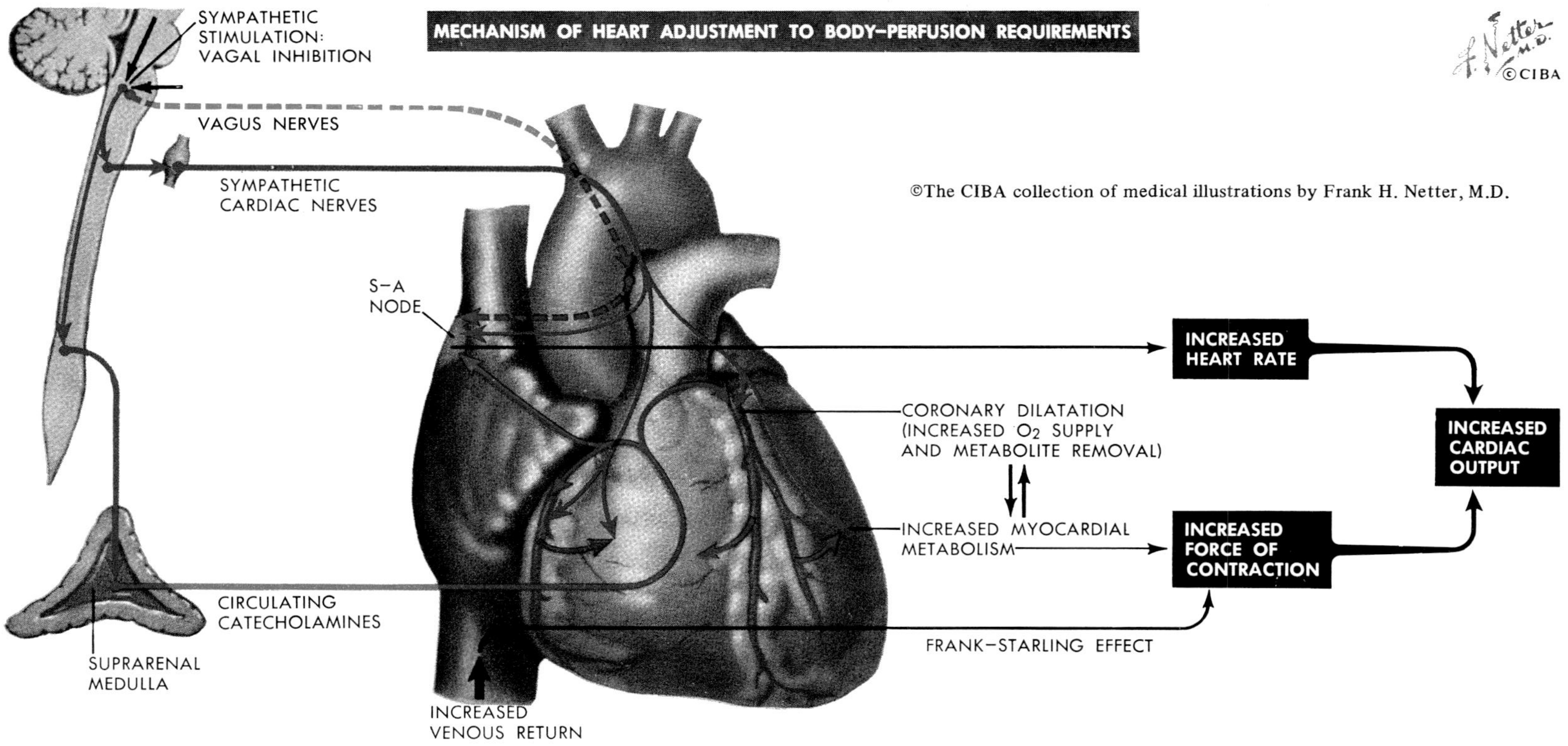

MECHANISM OF HEART ADJUSTMENT TO BODY-PERFUSION REQUIREMENTS

SYMPATHETIC
STIMULATION:
VAGAL INHIBITION

SYMPATHETIC
STIMULATION:
VAGAL INHIBITION

VAGUS NERVES

SYMPATHETIC
CARDIAC NERVES

SUPRARENAL
MEDULLA

CIRCULATING
CATECHOLAMINES

S–A
NODE

INCREASED
VENOUS RETURN

FRANK–STARLING EFFECT

INCREASED MYOCARDIAL
METABOLISM

CORONARY DILATATION
(INCREASED O₂ SUPPLY
AND METABOLITE REMOVAL)

INCREASED
FORCE OF
CONTRACTION

INCREASED
HEART RATE

INCREASED
CARDIAC
OUTPUT

© The CIBA collection of medical illustrations by Frank H. Netter, M.D.

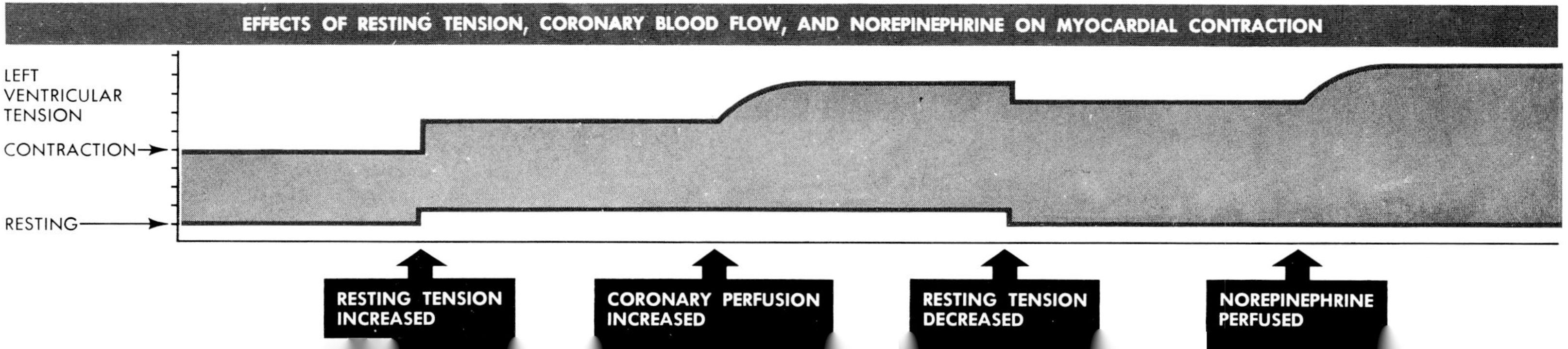

EFFECTS OF RESTING TENSION, CORONARY BLOOD FLOW, AND NOREPINEPHRINE ON MYOCARDIAL CONTRACTION

LEFT
VENTRICULAR
TENSION

CONTRACTION

RESTING

RESTING TENSION
INCREASED

CORONARY PERFUSION
INCREASED

RESTING TENSION
DECREASED

NOREPINEPHRINE
PERFUSED

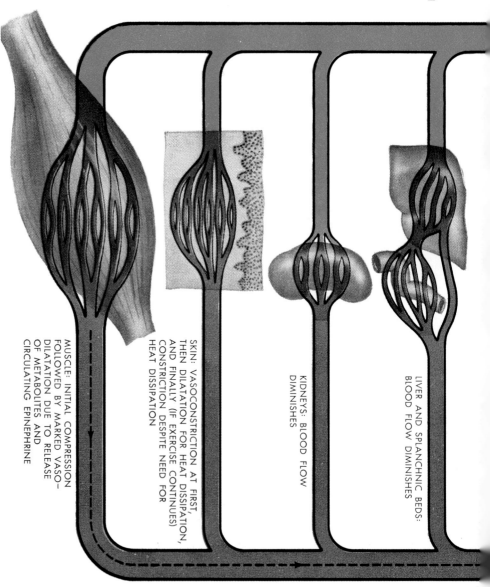

INCREASED
RATE OF
CONTRACTION

INCREASED
FORCE OF
CONTRACTION

MUSCLE: INITIAL COMPRESSION
FOLLOWED BY MARKED VASO-
DILATATION DUE TO RELEASE
OF METABOLITES AND
CIRCULATING EPINEPHRINE

SKIN: VASOCONSTRICTION AT FIRST,
THEN DILATATION FOR HEAT DISSIPATION,
AND FINALLY (IF EXERCISE CONTINUES)
CONSTRICTION DESPITE NEED FOR
HEAT DISSIPATION

KIDNEYS: BLOOD FLOW
DIMINISHES

LIVER AND SPLANCHNIC BEDS:
BLOOD FLOW DIMINISHES

Plate 3

CIRCULATORY RESPONSE TO EXERCISE

©The CIBA collection of medical illustrations by Frank H. Netter, M.D.

©CIBA

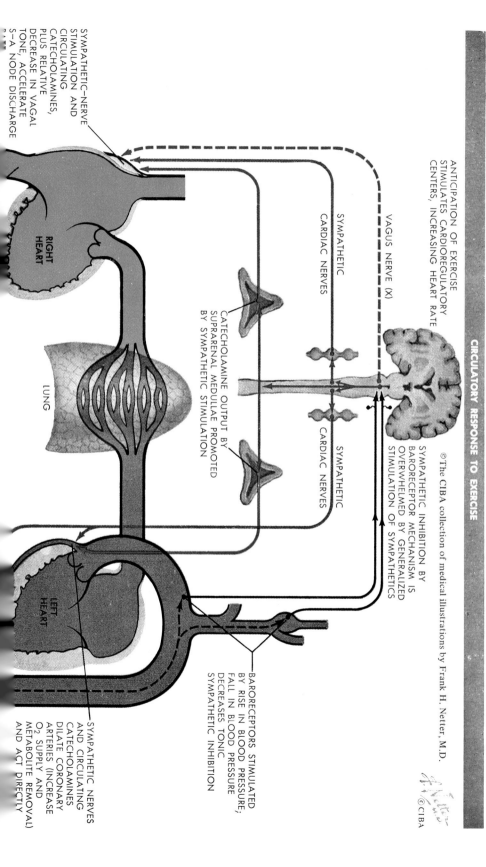

ANTICIPATION OF EXERCISE
STIMULATES CARDIOREGULATORY
CENTERS, INCREASING HEART RATE

SYMPATHETIC INHIBITION BY
BARORECEPTOR MECHANISM IS
OVERWHELMED BY GENERALIZED
STIMULATION OF SYMPATHETICS

VAGUS NERVE (X)

SYMPATHETIC
CARDIAC NERVES

SYMPATHETIC
CARDIAC NERVES

CATECHOLAMINE OUTPUT BY
SUPRARENAL MEDULLAE PROMOTED
BY SYMPATHETIC STIMULATION

SYMPATHETIC–NERVE
STIMULATION AND
CIRCULATING
CATECHOLAMINES,
PLUS RELATIVE
DECREASE IN VAGAL
TONE, ACCELERATE
S–A NODE DISCHARGE

RIGHT
HEART

LUNG

LEFT
HEART

BARORECEPTORS STIMULATED
BY RISE IN BLOOD PRESSURE;
FALL IN BLOOD PRESSURE
DECREASES TONIC
SYMPATHETIC INHIBITION

SYMPATHETIC NERVES
AND CIRCULATING
CATECHOLAMINES
DILATE CORONARY
ARTERIES (INCREASE
O₂ SUPPLY AND
METABOLITE REMOVAL)
AND ACT DIRECTLY

(b) a regional redistribution of blood, (c) an increase in heart rate, (d) an increase in blood pressure, (e) a decrease in total peripheral resistance and (f) an increase in cardiac output.

Circulatory response to exercise is presented in Plate 3.

While there is an increase in release of catecholamines during exercise, there is little or no change in endogenous levels of norepinephrine. The increased sympathetic activity accelerates the rate of synthesis of norepinephrine. Thus the increase in the rate of replenishment keeps pace with the rate of release and consequently, there is only slight or no reduction in catecholamine content of tissue.

LONG TERM CONTROL OF BLOOD PRESSURE

Nervous regulation of arterial blood pressure is very important in acute conditions such as changes in posture, hemorrhage or exercise. However, when blood pressure remains elevated for several days, the presso receptor adapts to protect. Therefore, in long term regulation of arterial pressure, nervous control has a limited usefulness. In the long term regulation a significant role is played by the kidney which acts both as an endocrine and as an excretory organ. Both these systems are semi-independent. The control of renal artery tone and the innervation of juxtaglomerular apparatus by the sympathetic nervous system allows them on occasion to operate synergistically.

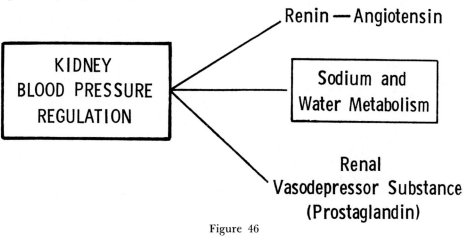

Figure 46

Figure 47. *Schematic Representation of the Mechanism of the Control of Volume by renin-angiotension-aldosterone System.*

Loss of sodium or decrease in plasma volume leading to decrease in renal blood flow stimulates an increase of renin and a rise in plasma angiotension concentration. This in turn would cause secretion of adlosterone which would act directly on distal renal tubules to bring about the retention of sodium and water in exchange for potassium anion and hydrogen ion. The consequent sodium retention causes expansion of plasma volume; cardiac output would thereby increase and blood pressure would rise to a level to restore the kidney perfusion.

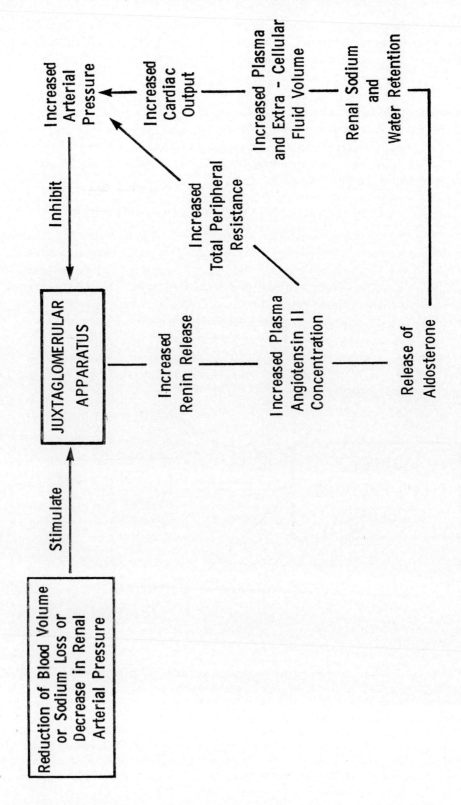

The kidney is critical in the long term control of blood pressure. It influences the blood pressure by three different mechanisms (Fig. 46). It regulates the blood pressure by controlling the fluid volume of the body. It does this through its control of salt and water metabolism. When blood pressure is increased from 100 to 200 mm Hg, the kidney increases the urinary output of both salt and water approximately six fold. On the other hand when blood pressure falls too low the extracellular fluid volume rises and restores the blood pressure (Fig. 47).

In addition to the extrinsic mechanism which is mediated through aldosterone, the kidney appears to have intrinsic mechanisms for controlling sodium and water excretion. It seems that transport of sodium and water across the renal tubules is influenced by a neural mechanism as well as by an unknown renal hormone other than renin. Thus the kidney has the ability to override extrinsic factors and by its effect on extracellular volume may, quite independently modulate systemic blood pressure.

The various factors (neural as well as humoral) controlling the blood pressure are depicted in Figure 48.

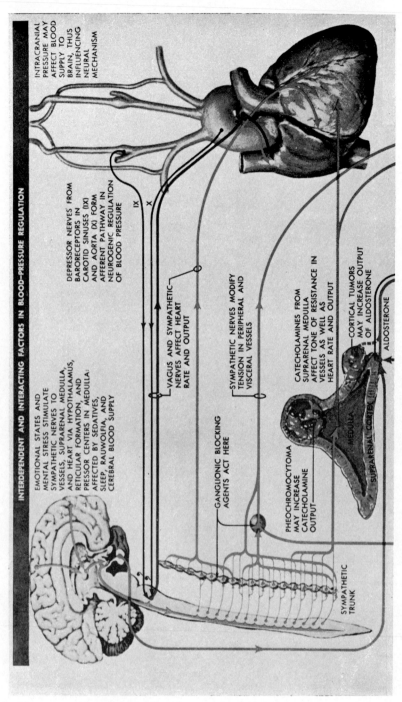

Figure 48. *Schematic Representation of the Factors Regulating Arterial Blood Pressure.*
There are at least four different methods by which arterial pressure is normally regulated. They are (1) the neural, (2) the endocrine, (3) the renal and (4) the cardiovascular. Although each of these factors can function independently, in life they act interdendently and work in concert.

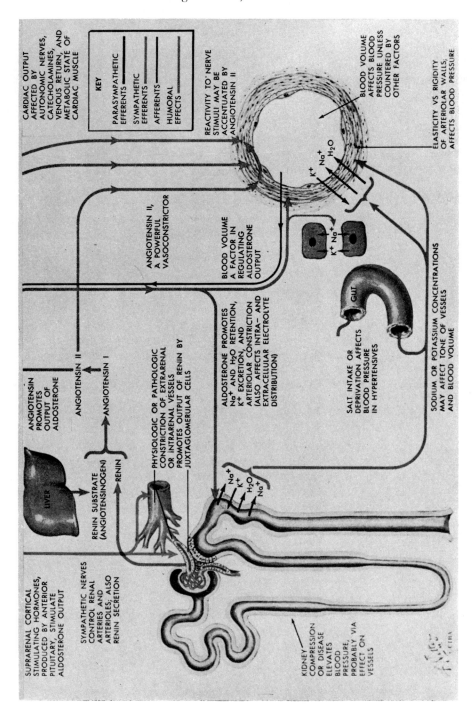

CHAPTER IX

RENIN AND ANGIOTENSIN SYSTEM

IN 1898, TIGERSTEDT and Bergman observed a prolonged rise of arterial pressure after intravenous injection of extracts of kidney cortex and gave the name renin to the responsible substance. Subsequently, it was found that renin is a proteolytic enzyme, and is synthesized in the vascular pole of the renal glomerulus of the kidney. These juxtaglomerular cells are specialized myoepithelial cells surrounding the afferent arterioles and respond to a decrease in stretch as a result of reduced perfusion pressure and renal blood flow by releasing renin. When there is a fall in mean arterial pressure, blood flow to the kidney is decreased. This decrease in intrarenal blood flow might be sensed by the juxtaglomerular cells as a decrease in the stretch exerted on afferent arteriolar walls; these cells would then release an increased renin secretion, within renal circulation (Plate 5). Just how reduced intrarenal blood pressure evokes the secretion of renin is not known. Some believe that it is the decreased pulse pressure rather than the decreased mean pressure that is responsible. Renin has no pressor activity, but requires the presence of an additional plasma factor to raise the blood pressure.

After release into the blood stream, renin acts on a plasma alpha-2-globulin substrate to yield a decapeptide angiotensin I. This substance is pharmacologically inert. The decapeptide interacts with converting enzymes to yield the active octapeptide angiotensin II. Angiotensinase, a normal constituent of the blood is capable of quickly inactivating angiotensin II (Plate 4).

Angiotensin II is one of the most powerful pressor agents known, acting through complex mechanisms involving central and peripheral nervous system (Fig. 49). It causes depolarization and contraction of arterial smooth muscle primarily by direct actions on the muscle cell. The effect on venous smooth muscle is variable. Angiotensin II exerts positive inotropic effect on isolated cardiac tissue, but its effects on the intact heart are not striking, perhaps because of its marked vasoconstrictor action on coronary arteries resulting in decreased myocardial blood flow. Angiotensin II also has the ability to activate the sympathetic nervous system (Fig. 50). It causes re-

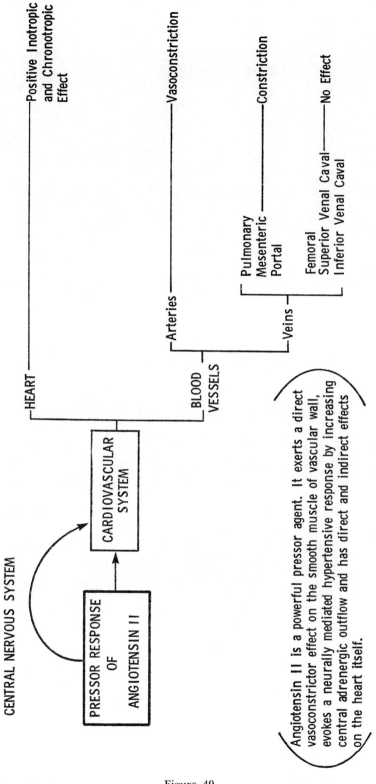

Figure 49

lease of catecholamines from its storage site (Feldberg and Lewis, 1964; Peach *et al.,* 1966; Robinson, 1967). McCubbin and Page (1963) have reported that angiotensin potentiated responses to agents and mechanical procedures which stimulated the sympathetic nervous system. This potentiating effect on sympathetic stimuli by angiotensin is probably due to an impairment of uptake into the adrenergic neuron (Peach *et al.,* 1969), and/or facilitation of neurally elicited released catecholamines (Zimmerman *et al.,* 1972). It has a striking stimulatory effect on catecholamine biosynthesis (Roth, 1972).

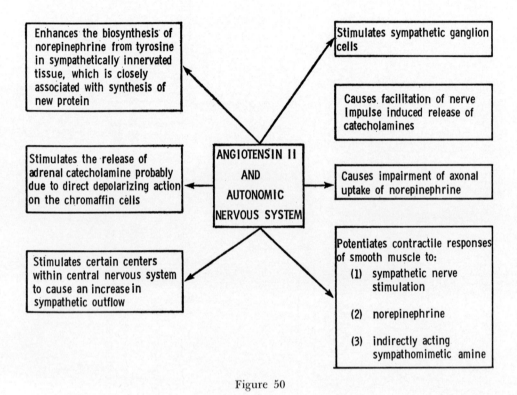

Figure 50

Angiotensin also stimulates the zona glomerulosa of the adrenal cortex to increase production and release of aldosterone. It stimulates not only the synthesis of aldosterone, but also the aldosterone precursor corticosterone. The primary action of plasma aldosterone is to increase the reabsorption of sodium by the renal tubules resulting in expansion of extracellular fluid volume and blood volume. Thus aldosterone increases both the sodium and the volume of water in the extracellular fluid. The expansion of the extracellular fluid helps to return the blood pressure to normal.

When the circulating blood volume is expanded, it would be sensed by the juxtaglomerular cells as increased stretch and would result in inhibition of renin formation and release. This would lead to a decrease in production and release of aldosterone and there would be an increase in sodium

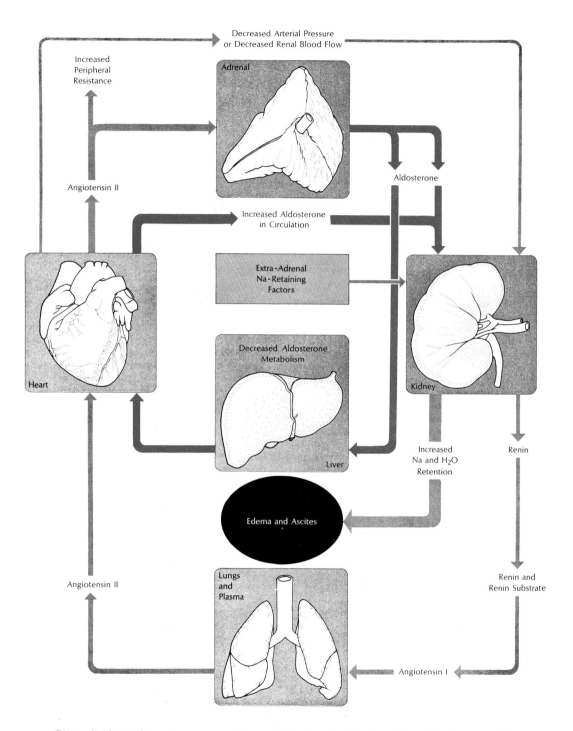

Plate 4 This schematic representation of factors leading to salt and water retention triggers renin release and activates the angiotensin-aldosterone system. In addition to direct effects on the kidney, alterations are present in circulatory dynamics in the liver and the periphery. The role of extra-adrenal Na-retaining factors is also indicated. Reproduced with permission from Davis J.O.: Hospital Practice.

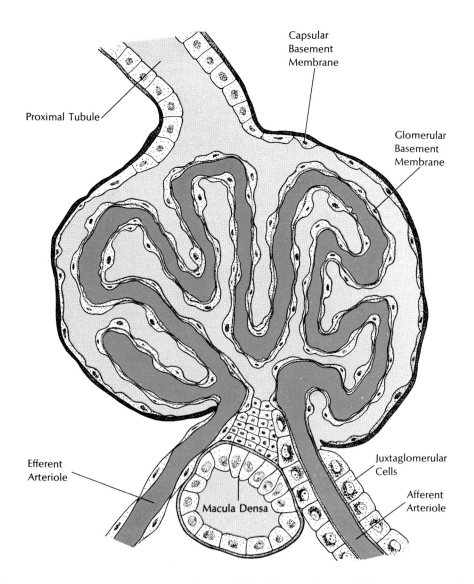

Plate 5 In this drawing of juxtaglomerular (JG) cells and the macula densa, one sees the anatomic relationships critical to many of the pathophysiologic events involved in the retention of sodium and water in congestive heart failure. Note the relationship of the JG cells to the lumen of the afferent arteriole into which they secrete renin and the proximity of the macula densa to the JG cells, suggesting its role in signaling renin release. Reproduced with permission from Davis J.O.: Hospital Practice.

Baroreceptor Hypothesis

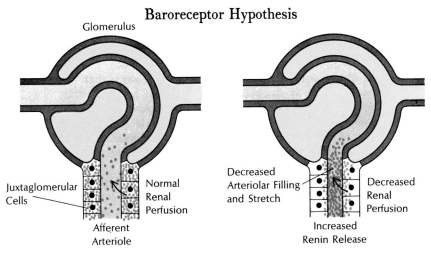

Glomerulus

Juxtaglomerular Cells

Normal Renal Perfusion

Afferent Arteriole

Decreased Arteriolar Filling and Stretch

Decreased Renal Perfusion

Increased Renin Release

Macula Densa Hypothesis

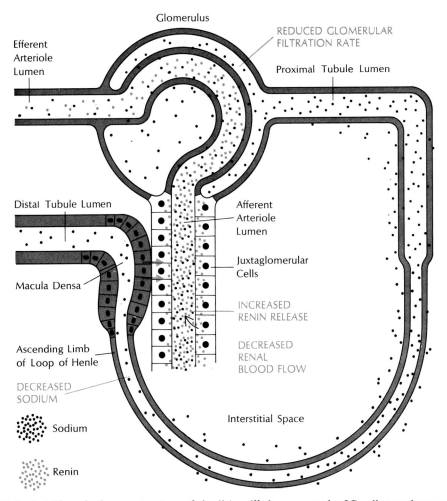

Glomerulus

Efferent Arteriole Lumen

REDUCED GLOMERULAR FILTRATION RATE

Proximal Tubule Lumen

Distal Tubule Lumen

Afferent Arteriole Lumen

Juxtaglomerular Cells

Macula Densa

INCREASED RENIN RELEASE

DECREASED RENAL BLOOD FLOW

Ascending Limb of Loop of Henle

DECREASED SODIUM

Interstitial Space

Sodium

Renin

Plate 6 Although the exact nature of the "signal" that causes the JG cells to release renin is not fully understood, two theories with variations provide the most widely accepted explanations. The baroreceptor theory postulates that the decreased renal perfusion occurs in association with a known marked reduction of renal blood flow in heart failure and results in incomplete filling at the level of the renal arterioles. This leads to decreased "stretch" in the JG cells and provides the signal for renin elaboration. An alternate hypothesis, the macula densa theory, suggests that as a result of reduced glomerular filtration, the sodium load reaching the distal tubule is reduced. This reduction is sensed by the macula densa, which is in close proximity to the JG cells and, possibly through the action of a local hormone (double arrow), signals them to secrete renin. Reproduced with permission from Davis J.O.: Hospital Practice.

excretion up to the point at which expanded extracellular fluid volume returned to normal. Thus, through a feedback mechanism, the kidneys respond to a decrease in mean arterial pressure by utilizing a humoral mechanism to regulate the blood pressure and blood volume.

RENIN SECRETION AND MACULA DENSA HYPOTHESIS

Another theoretical scheme of the events leading to the increased release of renin has been postulated (Plate 6). This theory suggests that the macula densa—the special staining cells of the distal tubular epithelium lying in close apposition to the juxtaglomerular cells—plays a pivotal role. When, as a result of reduced glomerular filtration, the sodium load reaching the distal tubule is reduced, the macula densa cells are activated to trigger release of renin by the juxtaglomerular cells, perhaps by the mediation of a local hormone.

Support for this concept comes from the morphologic observations that establish not only the proximity of the macula densa to the juxtaglomerular complex but also the presence of projections of macula densa cells toward the juxtaglomerular cells.

Regardless of the precise mechanism of renin release, it is clear that events leading to sodium retention are initiated by secretion of renin by the juxtaglomerular cells. Renin is secreted into the lumen of the renal afferent arterioles and thence enters the general circulation where the plasma renin levels are elevated.

RENIN SECRETION AND SYMPATHETIC NERVOUS SYSTEM

It is well known that when sympathetic fibers innervating the kidney are stimulated or catecholamines are administered, there is an increase in renin secretion. Furthermore, the addition of epinephrine in a suspension of kidney cells enhances the net renin production. These observations suggest that catecholamines stimulate renin production.

Since addition of cyclic AMP stimulates net renin production in renal cell suspension it is possible that cyclic AMP may be the intracellular mediator of the renin-stimulating action of catecholamines. Thus sodium loss, blood loss and sequestration of venous blood stimulate reflex sympathetic nervous system thereby increasing the renin secretion.

RENIN SECRETION AND ANGIOTENSIN

Plasma concentration of angiotensin can also affect the renin production and release. For example when angiotensin is administered, it causes a fall in renin production *in vivo*. Likewise, the infusion of angiotensin into one renal artery diminishes renin production by that kidney and addition of angiotensin inhibits net renin production by a suspension of kidney cells. Thus increase in plasma angiotensin diminishes the formation of renin which in turn inhibits further generation of angiotensin.

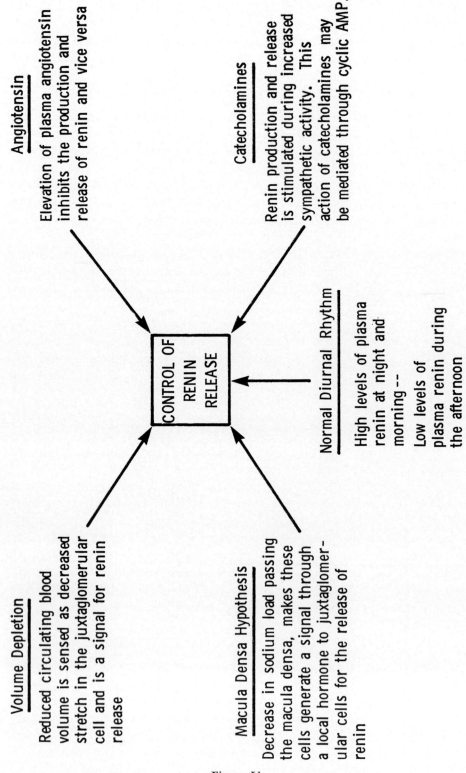

Angiotensin

Elevation of plasma angiotensin inhibits the production and release of renin and vice versa

Catecholamines

Renin production and release is stimulated during increased sympathetic activity. This action of catecholamines may be mediated through cyclic AMP.

CONTROL OF RENIN RELEASE

Normal Diurnal Rhythm

High levels of plasma renin at night and morning--
Low levels of plasma renin during the afternoon

Volume Depletion

Reduced circulating blood volume is sensed as decreased stretch in the juxtaglomerular cell and is a signal for renin release

Macula Densa Hypothesis

Decrease in sodium load passing the macula densa, makes these cells generate a signal through a local hormone to juxtaglomerular cells for the release of renin

Figure 51

RENIN SECRETION AND DIURNAL VARIATION

In addition to these possible renin control mechanisms, normal diurnal rhythm influences the renin secretion. Thus, normal individuals have relatively high renin activity during the night and morning and lower levels during afternoon.

Factors controlling the renin release are presented in Figure 51.

FUNCTIONS OF THE RENIN-AGIOTENSIN SYSTEM

The role of the renin-angiotensin system in the body is not clearly defined. It is believed that this system has at least the following three functions:

1. It causes a release of aldosterone and thereby regulates the sodium balance.
2. It regulates the blood volume through its action on aldosterone release.
3. It regulates blood pressure through the action of angiotensin on blood volume and peripheral arteriolar resistance.

CHAPTER X

PROSTAGLANDINS

IN 1934 VON EULER isolated a lipid substance from the animal fluid and vesicular gland, which caused a fall in blood pressure when injected intravenously. Von Euler named this substance prostaglandin (PG) since this substance was abundantly present in the prostate gland. Elucidation of the structure of prostaglandin by Bergstrom and coworkers (1968) revealed that it was not a single substance, but a large family of closely related substances. All prostaglandins are 20 carbon hydroxy fatty acids with a cyclopentane ring. The three major groups of prostaglandins are E, F, and A, so named on the basis of their ring structure. The number in the subscript position indicates the degree of unsaturation in the side chains. Recently Corey and his co-workers have been successful in total chemical synthesis of all prostaglandins.

Prostaglandins are found in a wide variety of tissues such as lungs, kidney, brain, heart, stomach, liver, intestine, uterus, placenta, testicles, seminal vesicles and iris. They are also found in human seminal plasma. There is enough evidence to suggest that free unsaturated fatty acids such as dihomo-y-linolenic acid and arachidonic acid in the tissues are rapidly converted into prostaglandins. The rate limiting step appears to be the release of the fatty acids from their combined state in lipids such as phospholipids. They are released from tissue in response to various stimuli. On release, they are rapidly inactivated by enzymes in the lungs, kidney, and liver. Hence, the concentrations of circulating plasma prostaglandins are extremely low.

CARDIOVASCULAR ACTION

The effects of the prostaglandins on the cardiovascular system are complicated by differences among the prostaglandins and by species variations. Generally E and A prostaglandins are considered qualitatively alike whereas the F prostaglandins often are very different.

Heart

Prostaglandins exert positive inotropic and chronotropic effects on the

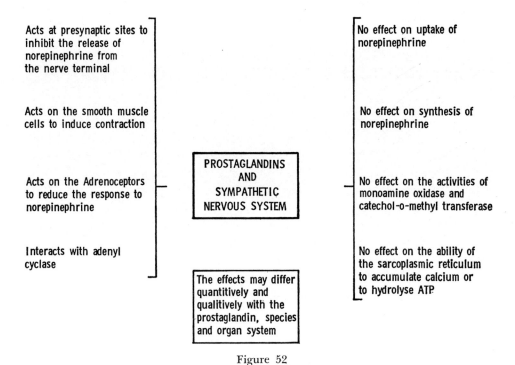

Figure 52

isolated heart. The cardiostimulatory responses to prostaglandins remain unaltered when β-adrenoceptors are blocked by propranolol and when catecholamine stores are depleted by prior treatment of animals with reserpine. This suggests that these effects of prostaglandins are not mediated through the release of catecholamines or through the stimulation of adrenoceptors (Bhagat *et al;* 1972). The effect may, therefore, be due to a direct effect on the muscle.

In the isolated atrial preparation, the cardiostimulatory effects of prostaglandins E_2 were found to be independent of the increase in calcium ion concentration in the bathing medium. However, when the calcium ion concentration in the bathing solution was decreased from 1.6mM to 0.8mM, the positive inotropic response was enhanced by twofold.

Prostaglandins E_1, F_1, and A_2 did not show any action on calcium binding, calcium uptake, or total ATPase activity of the cardiac sarcoplasmic reticulum (Bhagat *et al;* 1972).

Vascular Smooth Muscles

The prostaglandins E and A series exert a vasodilator action in almost all arterioles and thereby increase the regional blood flow and cause a fall in blood pressure. The vasodilator and hypotensive actions of prostaglandins E and prostaglandins A compound remain unaltered by vagotomy, sympathectomy, or by pretreatment with atropine, propranolol, and methysergide. Thus, the vasodilator actions of prostaglandins are direct on the vascular smooth muscle and are not mediated through stimulation of cholinergic or adrengic receptors or by histamine or serotonin release (Horton, 1969, Nakano, 1971). This vasodilator action is, however, reduced by norepinephrine, angiotensin and vasopressin (Horton, 1969). Prostaglandin F compounds, in contrast to E and A compounds, constrict arterioles and venules and decrease the regional blood flow.

Coronary circulation. Prostaglandins E and A increase in coronary blood and decrease in coronary resistance. The response is a direct vascular effect and is not primarily due to increased metabolic requirements of the myocardium, since in paced beta blocked preparation prostaglandins E_2 still caused 42 percent decrease in coronary vascular resistance (Higgin *et al;* 1971) Prostaglandins F_a has no effect.

Systemic circulation. The prostaglandins of A and E series cause a fall in blood pressure in proportion to the dose administered. Since prostaglandins of A series are not appreciably metabolized in the lungs and since prostaglandin E compounds are inactivated in the single circulation through the lungs, prostaglandins A compound exerts a greater hypotensive effect than prostaglandins E compound, when given intravenously.

The lowering of blood pressure after prostaglandins E and A is accompanied by an increase in cardiac output secondary to a reflex tachycardia so that peripheral resistance falls markedly. The hypotensive action is mediated primarily by mesenteric arteriolar dilatation; femoral and renal blood flow relatively is less affected. There is also constant rise in carotid blood flow during the fall in systemic blood pressure resulting from prostaglandins A indicating active cerebral vasodilation during systemic vasodilation.

In contrast to prostaglandins E and A, prostaglandins F compounds exerts a slight increase in systemic arterial pressure, cardiac output, myocardial contractility, and vascular resistance.

Renal prostaglandins and hypertension. The prostaglandins (PGE_2 and possibly PGA_2) are synthesized, stored and readily metabolized in the kidney. Whereas the prostaglandins are localized primarily in the inner medulla, the enzymes responsible for degradation are believed to be located in the outer medullary and cortical regions. The factors that control their release are unknown. It has been shown that Prostaglandin-like material is released during renal ischemia (McGiff *et al;* 1970), during infusion of norepinephrine (Fujimoto and Lockett, 1970), and during renal nerve stimulation (Durham and Zimmerman, 1970).

Lee *et al.* (1971) found that infusion of PGA, in the patients with essential hypertension at a rate of 0.5 to 1.01 $\mu g/kg$ body min. caused a marked rise in renal blood flow, natriuresis and increased urine flow without change in systemic blood pressure. The findings suggest that renal blood vessels are more sensitive to PGA than other blood vessels. When the infusion rate was increased to 5 to 10 $\mu g/kg$ body weight per min., blood pressure fell and renal blood flow, urine flow and sodium excretion returned to normal limits. Thus, the systemic hypotension induced by PGA negated its direct effect on renal blood flow and sodium excretion. Renal function was well maintained during lowering of blood pressure by PGA. Since the PGA compounds appear to be renal antihypertensive agents, Lee postulated that deficiency of renal prostaglandins could contribute to the pathogenesis of hypertension. In support of this concept, Somova & Dochev (1970) found that chronic renal hypertension in the rat was successfully treated with PGE_1 or PGE_2, (15 to 30 μg/kg intraperitoneally) daily for 30 days. However, elevated plasma angiotensinase activity was unaffected and there was rise in plasma renin.

Much work is needed, however, before prostaglandins can take a place in modern antihypertensive therapy.

The interaction of prostaglandin with sympathetic nervous system is shown in Figure 52.

CHAPTER XI

ADRENERGIC RECEPTORS

THE ADRENERGIC RECEPTORS are hypothetical parts of the effector cell that selectively receive molecules of norepinephrine and its
analogues. In 1905, Langley proposed that there are two types of tissue
receptors, excitatory and inhibitory and that response to epinephrine depends on the type of receptor with which it reacts. This hypothesis was
supported by Dale's studies in 1906. He found that when 0.5 mg of the
active principle of ergot was injected, an intravenous administration of
200 mg of epinephrine did not cause the usual rise of blood pressure in
the spinal cat. If another dose of epinephrine was given, the blood pressure

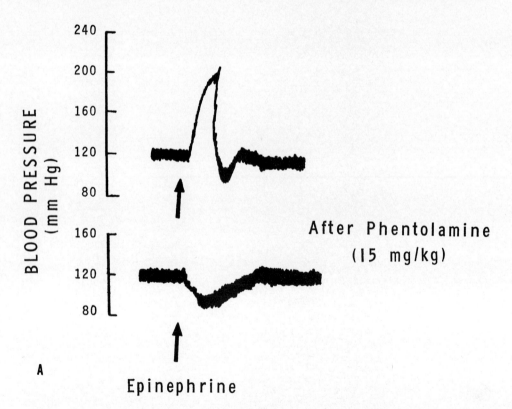

did fall (Fig. 53A). Although the constrictor action of epinephrine on the blood vessels was completely antagonized by ergotoxin, the cardiac stimulatory action of epinephrine still remained. Thus, these results suggested that there are at least two sites on which epinephrine can act, one of which was blocked by administration of active principle of ergot.

Classification of Adrenergic Receptors

It remained for Ahlquist (1948) to define clearly the concept of alpha and beta adrenergic receptors. He studied the effect of six closely related sympathomimetic amines on a variety of different systems and found differences in the order of responsiveness. In one case norepinephrine was the most active, while isoproterenol was least active. However, in other cases the order of potency was completely reversed, i.e. isoproterenol was the most active. On the basis of these findings, he postulated the existence of two types of receptors. Receptors which on stimulation cause excitatory responses are called alpha receptors. Those with an inhibitory response are called beta receptors. In terms of circulatory responses the cardiac stimulatory activity and vasodilation produced by sympathomimetic amines were classified as beta adrenergic responses, and vasoconstriction as alpha.

Although the adrenergic receptors have not been isolated chemically, it is believed that enzyme adenylcyclase in the cell membrane may represent at least a part of the receptor mechanism. Adenylcylase catalyzes the formation of cyclic 3'-5' adenosine monophosphate (cyclic AMP), and it appears that cyclic AMP mediates the effects of many hormones in the body, thus acting as a second messenger.

The support for this classification was derived from the studies with antagonists. In fact, the concept of classification of adrenergic receptors was not accepted until the discovery of dichloroisoproterenol (DCI), a derivative of isoproterenol. This drug blocked adrenergic stimulatory effects on the heart did not antagonize the vasoconstriction induced by sympathomimetic amines. Since DCI antagonized those effects of adrenergic stimulation which were not blocked by ergot and which were designated by Ahlquist as beta type, DCI was classified as beta adrenergic blocking agent.

Since the discovery of DCI, a large number of related compounds have

Figure 53 A

Effect of α-adrenergic blockade on the blood pressure response to epinephrine. A dog was anesthetized with pentobarbital and received 1 mg/kg atropine prior to the experiment to prevent reflex bradycardia. Injection of epinephrine caused a rise of blood pressure, which fell below control levels before returning to normal. The epinephrine activates both α and β receptors, but action on β-receptor is masked by the action on α-receptor. When phentalamine was injected the α-receptors were blocked. An injection of epinephrine could then activate only β-receptor, therefore it caused blood pressure fall. The change of the pressor response of injected epinephrine into a depressor response, is called the "epinephrine reversal."

been prepared and tested for beta blocking activities. They have certain advantages over DCI. They are more potent and, unlike DCI, they have no intrinsic sympathomimetic activity. For example, propranolol causes beta-adrenergic blockade without the side effect of excessive tachycardia. It is also several times more potent as a beta-blocking drug than DCI.

Specificity of β-Blocking Drugs

Unlike α-blocking agents, β-receptor-blocking drugs have a relatively high degree of specificity. For example, cardio-stimulatory response to nerve stimulation or to sympathomimetic amines is blocked by β-receptor-blocking drugs, whereas these antagonists do not block the response to other cardio-stimulants, such as calcium, theophylline or digoxin. Likewise, whereas vasodilation caused by isoproterenol is antagonized, vasodilation in response to acetylcholine, nitroglycerine and histamine remains unaltered.

CLASSIFICATION OF RECEPTORS

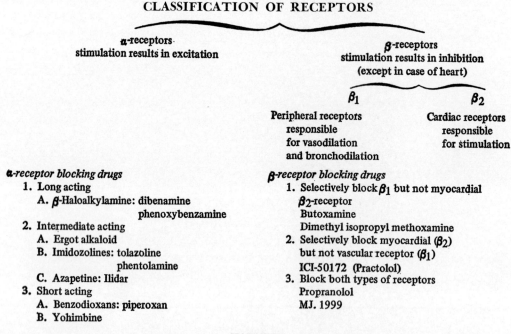

α-receptors stimulation results in excitation	β-receptors stimulation results in inhibition (except in case of heart)	
	β_1	β_2
	Peripheral receptors responsible for vasodilation and bronchodilation	Cardiac receptors responsible for stimulation

α-receptor blocking drugs
1. Long acting
   A. β-Haloalkylamine: dibenamine
      phenoxybenzamine
2. Intermediate acting
   A. Ergot alkaloid
   B. Imidozolines: tolazoline
      phentolamine
   C. Azapetine: Ilidar
3. Short acting
   A. Benzodioxans: piperoxan
   B. Yohimbine

β-receptor blocking drugs
1. Selectively block β_1 but not myocardial β_2-receptor
   Butoxamine
   Dimethyl isopropyl methoxamine
2. Selectively block myocardial (β_2) but not vascular receptor (β_1)
   ICI-50172 (Practolol)
3. Block both types of receptors
   Propranolol
   MJ. 1999

TABLE VI

Classification of β-Receptors

Further development of beta-adrenoceptors agonists and antagonists have indicated that there are differences in β-receptors of different tissues. For example, heart receptors are considered beta on the basis of selective block-ade with propranolol, but norepinephrine exerts a stronger action on the beta-adrenoceptors of the heart causing an increase in both the rate and force of contraction, whereas it is very weak agonist on the beta receptors of blood vesels in skeletal muscles. On the basis of such findings, it has been suggested that beta-adrenoceptors might be classified as at least two types (Lands and Brown, 1964; Lands *et al.*, 1967). The beta$_1$ adrenoceptors include those in the peripheral system responsible for vasodilation, bronchodilation and uterine relaxation. The beta$_2$ adrenoceptors include those in the heart (and gut?). A classification of adrenergic receptors is given in Table VI. The evidence for this division is the discovery of selective beta-blocking agents. For example, N-isopropylmethoxamine and butoxamine antagonize peripheral vasodilation response to isoproterenol without affecting the cardiac response (Levy, 1964, 1966a,b, 1967). On the other hand, a more recently developed compound, 1C1-50172 (2-hydroxy-3-isopropyla-minopropoxy-acetanilid; practolol) a cardioselective β_2-blocker, blocks only the β_2-receptors of the heart without affecting those of vascular smooth muscle (Dunlop and Shanks, 1968). Comparison of the selected β-adrenergic blocking drugs is presented in Table VII.

TABLE VII

Comparison of Selected β-adrenergic Blocking Drugs

| | Receptor Blockade | | | | |
	β_1 Receptor Vascular	β_2 Receptors Cardiac	Local Anesthetic Effect	Intrinsic Sympathomimetic Activity	Cardiac Catecholamines After Chronic Administration* (% of control)
Drug					
Alprenolol	+	+	+	+ +	138
Propranolol	+	+	+	—	112
Practolol	—	+	—	+	84
Satalol	+	+	—	—	. . .
Oxprenolol	+	+	+	+ +	98

*10 mg/kg of drug was injected subcutaneously daily for about 11 days, in rats.

CIRCULATORY SYSTEM

The distribution of receptors, and the respective effector responses as they concern circulatory system are given in Table VIII. When a cardiac sympathetic nerve is stimulated, it increases heart rate, force of atrial and ventricular contraction, and activation of glycogenolysis. After propranolol, there is complete or partial inhibition of the effects of sympathetic nerve stimulation or of intravenous injections of catecholamine on the heart. Whereas tachycardia in response to adrenergic stimulation is antagonized after propranolol, it does not inhibit the reflex bradycardia elicited by sympathomimetic amines such as phenylephrine or methoxamine. Phenoxybenzamine, phentolamine and other α-receptor adrenergic blocking drugs do not block the effects of cardiac sympathetic nerve stimulation. Therefore, sympathetic stimulation of cardiac activity is mediated by β_2-receptors. Govier (1968) has suggested the possibility of α-receptors in the heart. Assuming that α-receptors do exist in the myocardium, their functional significance may be of minor importance as compared to β_2-receptors. Effects of blockade of myocardial adrenergic receptors are presented in (Table IX, Fig. 53B).

TABLE VIII

The Response of Circulatory System to Adrenergic Stimulation

Organ	Response	Receptor
Heart		
Sinoatrial node rate	Increased	β_2
Atrioventricular conduction	Increased	β_2
Contractility of ventricular myocardium	Increased	β_2
Vasculature		
(a) *Arteries*		
skin, mesenteric, and renal	Constriction	α
*coronary	Dilation	β_1 (Predominant)
	Constriction	α
skeletal	Dilation	β_1
(b) *Vein*	Constriction	α

α-Receptor and β_2 receptor stimulation results in excitatory response.

β_1-Receptor stimulation result in inhibitory responses.

*Under normal conditions coronary dilatation is produced by the increased local myocardial oxygen requirement resulting from the direct positive inotropic and chronotropic effect of catecholamines on the myocardium (indirect). Isoproterenol can cause vasodilation due to direct stimulation of β_1 receptors which can be blocked by propranolol. Norepinephrine can cause coronary constriction, which could be blocked by the alpha blocking drug phentolamine. Alpha receptor activity is of much less degree than in peripheral vasculature.

TABLE IX

RESULTS OF BLOCKADE OF CARDIAC β_2-ADRENOCEPTOR

Blockade of cardiac β_2-adrenoreceptor may result in a decrease in
1. Heart beat.
2. Cardiac output.
3. Stroke volume.
4. Stroke work.
5. Effect of exercise on heart rate and cardiac output.

The degree of these hemodynamic effects depends on
1. Dose of the drug.
2. Potency of the drug.
3. Degree of sympathetic tone present prior to administration of drug.

RECEPTORS IN BLOOD VESSELS

The distribution of adrenergic receptors in the blood vessels is more complex.

Arteries

The arteries are the major resistance vessels, and are innervated mainly by sympathetic nerves. The stimulation of these nerves on administration of norepinephrine causes vasoconstriction, and the primary effect of sympathetic nerve stimulation is determined in part by the number and distribution of these receptors. This vasoconstriction is antagonized by α-receptor blocking drugs such as phenoxybenzamine and phentolamine. In contrast, when isoproterenol is injected it shows very little effect and does not cause vasoconstriction. Furthermore, beta adrenergic blocking drugs such as propranolol fail to antagonize sympathetically induced vasoconstriction. Thus, vasoconstriction of the resistance vessels is mediated by α-receptors. α-Adrenoreceptor activity is prominent in the precapillary vessels of most of the vessel.

Coronary Arteries

Adrenergic stimulation to the heart results in an increased coronary blood flow. It is mostly due to enhanced myocardial contractility and metabolism. Adrenergic receptors in the smooth muscles of coronary blood vessels have

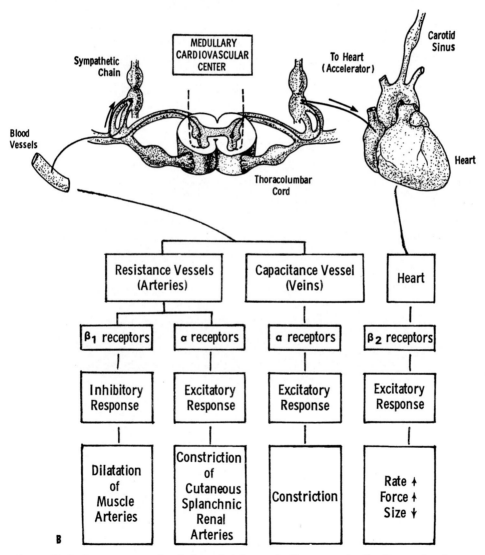

Figure 53 B. Response to stimulation of Adrenergic Receptors in Cardiovascular System

been the subject of great controversy. Bohr (1967) has demonstrated that isolated helical strips of a coronary vascular smooth muscle segment, dilated in response to isoproterenol, norepinephrine and epinephrine. After β-adrenergic blockade with propranolol, isolated artery strips showed a constrictor response to these agonists suggesting the presence of α-receptors. Recently, Malindzak *et al.*, (1972) injected these drugs directly into coronary artery of an anesthesized dog and measured the response immediately; the systemic effects and reflexes on the coronary blood flow were thereby eliminated. They found an increase in coronary blood flow and a decrease in coronary artery resistance in response to intra-arterial injection of epinephrine, norepinephrine and phenylephrine, indicating a vasodilation. Following beta blockade by propranolol, there was an increase in coronary artery resistance in response to the intracoronary injection of epinephrine, norepinephrine and phenylephrine suggesting vasoconstriction. On the basis of these findings they concluded that coronary artery has both β and α receptors. Norepinephrine and epinephrine, etc., increase coronary blood flow by activating β_1 dilator receptors. In the coronary vasculature, these drugs decrease coronary blood flow by activating alpha constrictor receptors (in coronary vasculature) after being unmasked by propranolol.

Arteries in Skeletal Muscle

The β-receptors in the blood vessels of the skeletal muscle are not usually considered to be innervated. Recently, Oberg and Rosell have reported that stimulation of the sympathetic nerves to adipose tissue causes vasodilation in dogs. The response is antagonized by propranolol. Likewise, in the gracilis muscle of the dog, stimulation of sympathetic nerves produce vasodilation through β-adrenergic receptors.

Thus, it appears that sympathetic nerves probably mediate adrenergic vasodilation in skeletal muscle and are capable of effecting reduction in systemic vascular resistance and a fall of mean arterial blood pressure.

Veins

Veins are innervated by the sympathetic nerves, which upon stimulation cause constriction. The venoconstriction is mediated through α-receptors.

PHYSIOLOGICAL SIGNIFICANCE OF β-RECEPTORS

Important information regarding the significance of adrenergic receptors has been obtained from the studies of the response to exercise (Fig. 54). Increase in sympathetic nervous activity associated with exercise causes release of catecholamines from the sympathetic nerve endings as well as from suprarenal medulla. This brings about a sequence of cardiovascular events that represents a combination of effects produced by participation of all types of adrenergic receptors. There is a cardiac stimulation which is mediated through the stimulation of β_2-adrenergic receptors, arteriolar

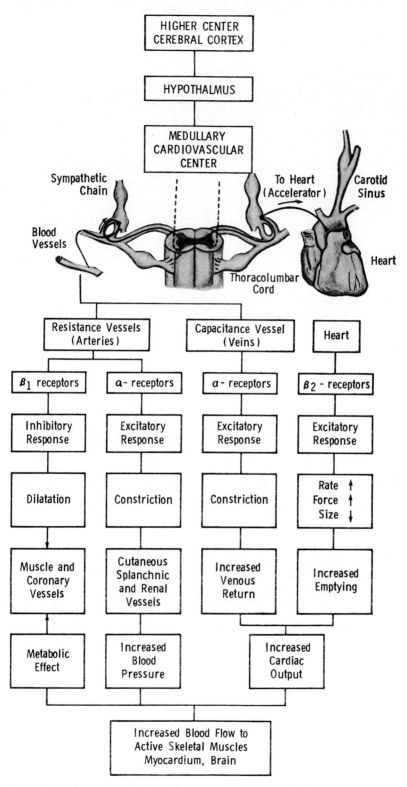

Figure 54. Schematic representation of the role of sympathetic nervous system in the circulatory response to exercise.

vasoconstriction mediated through the stimulation of α-receptor in liver, renal and splanchnic areas and β_1 mediated vasodilation in skeletal muscle.

The net results of the exercise are:

1. an increase in heart rate
2. an increase in blood pressure
3. a decrease in total peripheral resistance
4. an increase in cardiac output
5. reduced blood flow to *non-vital* organs

Exercise-induced tachycardia is the result of (1) decreased vagal activity to the S-A node of the heart and (2) enhanced sympathetic activity to the S-A node. Beta adrenergic blocking drugs antagonize only the effects of increased sympathetic nervous activity. In racing greyhounds, for example, the tachycardia resulting during the race was only partially inhibited by beta blocking drugs. In the greyhound with denervated heart, acceleration of the heart rate during the race was completely antagonized by propranolol. It seems that acceleration of the heart rate in the greyhound with innervated heart, pretreated with beta blocking drug, was mainly due to inhibition of vagal activity and therefore propranolol failed to block it completely. In contrast, in dogs with denervated hearts, exercise-induced tachycardia was due entirely to circulating catecholamines and was therefore antagonized by propranolol.

There is no parasympathetic nerve supply to the ventricles. Therefore, reflex inhibition of vagal activity does not enhance the ventricular contractile activity. This is in contrast to effect of vagal inhibition on S-A node whch results in increased firing. The role of the parasympathetic nervous system in ventricular contraction is therefore not as great as that of the sympathetic system. Propranolol is quite effective therefore in depressing the increase in ventricular activity produced by exercise.

The exercise-induced increase in cardiac output is mainly due to increased activity of the sympathetic nervous system and is therefore antagonized by block of Beta receptors in the ventricular myocardium. The effects of exercise on the cardiovascular system are depicted in Figure 54.

HYPERTENSION

Beta adrenergic blockade is used in the treatment of a wide variety of cardiovascular diseases (Table X). Chronic oral administration of propranolol reduces arterial pressure without producing orthostatic hypo-

TABLE X

Usefulness of β-blockade in cardiac diseases

β-blockade is of value where sympathetic activity is inappropriate and contributing significantly to the patient's conditions. It is being used in:

1. Angina pectoris
2. Arrhythmias
3. Hypertension
4. Hypertrophic obstructive cardiomyopathy
5. Hyperkinetic heart syndrome

tension. The reduction in arterial pressure is due to a depresion of cardiac output rather than a decrease in peripheral vascular resistance. It is therefore effective in patients with mild to moderate hypertension. Short term oral therapy or intravenous administration of propranolol is ineffective.

Complications of Beta Adrenergic Therapy

The most serious complications of propranolol therapy are the natural consequences of its action as a blocker of the beta adrenergic receptors. Beta blockade results in a reduction in myocardial contractility, and the condition of any patient who is dependent upon his sympathetic nervous system to maintain circulatory compensation, may deteriorate following β-blockade. Deaths associated with propranolol have occurred in patients in whom myocardial function was already impaired by acute myocardial infarction, congestive heart failure, or a severe dysrhythmia. Hypotension, hypoglycemia, severe bradycardia, and, rarely, complete heart block have also been reported as complications. A history of bronchial asthma is an indication for caution in the use of propranolol since blockade of beta adrenergic receptors prevents adrenergic bronchodilatation and thereby leaves the vagal effects on the bronchial tree unopposed. However, practolol might be of value in asthmatic patients since it is "cardioselective" and does not block bronchial beta adrenergic receptors. Propranolol should also be avoided in patients being treated with mono-amine-oxidase inhibitors or other adrenergic-augmenting psychotropic drugs. The other side effects of propranolol administration are infrequent and mild and rarely necessitate discontinuation of therapy.

Chapter XII

ACTIONS OF NOREPINEPHRINE, EPINEPHRINE AND OTHER AMINES ON THE CARDIOVASCULAR SYSTEM

SYMPATHOMIMETIC AMINES DIFFER greatly in their cardiac and peripheral action and consequently, in their overall effect on the cardiovascular system. This difference is probably due to their different potency on various adrenergic receptors (Table XI). They are classified into three groups, Group I, drugs which stimulate the myocardium and may elevate the blood pressure, e.g. norepinephrine and epinephrine; Group 2, drugs

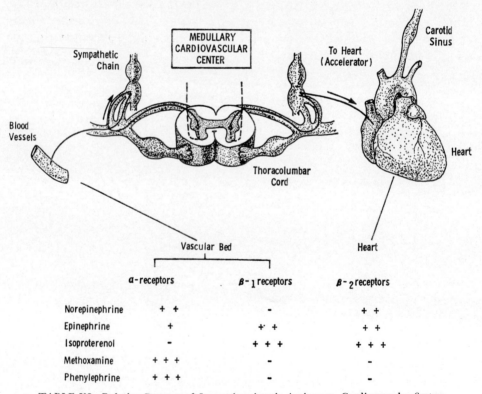

	α-receptors	β-1 receptors	β-2 receptors
Norepinephrine	+ +	-	+ +
Epinephrine	+	+ +	+ +
Isoproterenol	-	+ + +	+ + +
Methoxamine	+ + +	-	-
Phenylephrine	+ + +	-	-

TABLE XI   Relative Potency of Sympathomimetic Amines on Cardiovascular System

which stimulate the myocardium but cause a fall in blood pressure, e.g. isoproterenol; and Group 3, drugs which have little effect on the myocardium but elevate blood pressure, e.g. phenylephrine and methoxamine.

Norepinephrine and epinephrine stimulate both alpha and beta receptors. In arterioles, epinephrine has greater affinity for beta receptors causing vasodilation in low concentrations. Larger amounts of epinephrine result in alpha receptor stimulation as well, and the dominant effect is vasoconstriction. Norepinephrine has a greater affinity for alpha receptors, causing only vasoconstriction of blood vessels. In the heart, both catecholamines strongly stimulate the myocardial $beta_2$ receptors. Dopamine is similar in its action to norepinephrine with the additional property that it causes renal and splanchnic vasodilation by a separate receptor mechanism. Methoxamine and phenylephrine stimulate only alpha receptors and are purely vasoconstrictive. Isoproterenol is a pure beta receptor activator and causes cardiac stimulation and vasodilation. (Netter has presented the actions of sympathomimetic amines in a simplified form).

GROUP 1

Norepinephrine

Norepinephrine (Fig. 55) has the following effects:

1. Norepinephrine acts on α-receptors in the vascular bed and causes an increase in peripheral resistance that leads to an increase in systolic, diastolic and mean arterial pressure due to vasoconstriction.
2. The rise in mean arterial pressure activates the baroreceptors. Increase in impulse discharge in the carotid sinus and aortic nerves stimulates the vagus nerve.
3. The overall sympathetic tone is diminished, while vagal tone is increased.
4. Heart rate may be decreased despite the moderate stimulation of the heart by direct action.
5. Cardiac output may not change or may decrease.
6. Peripheral blood flow may be decreased.

Epinephrine

Epinephrine (Fig. 56) has the following effects:

1. Epinephrine acts on both alpha and beta receptors in the vascular bed. In small doses, the effect of epinephrine on beta receptors may predominate, resulting in dilation in certain peripheral blood vessels, especially in skeletal muscles. Total peripheral resistance may fall, which may actually cause a fall in diastolic pressure.

Figure 55. Adapted from Frank H. Netter, M.D., CIBA collection of medical illustrations.

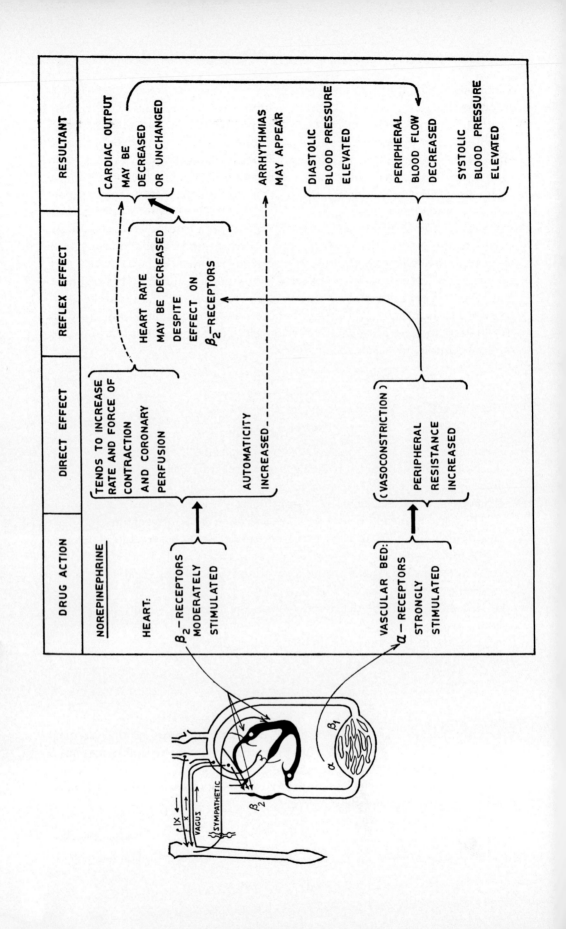

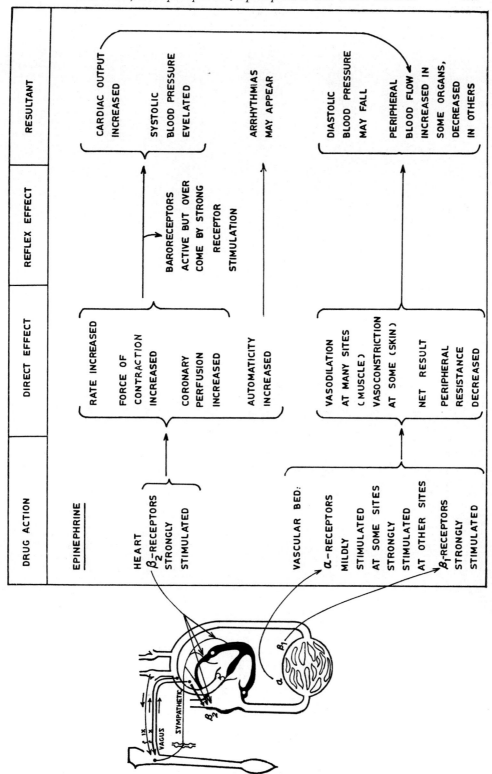

Figure 56. Adapted from Frank H. Netter, M.D., CIBA collection of medical illustrations.

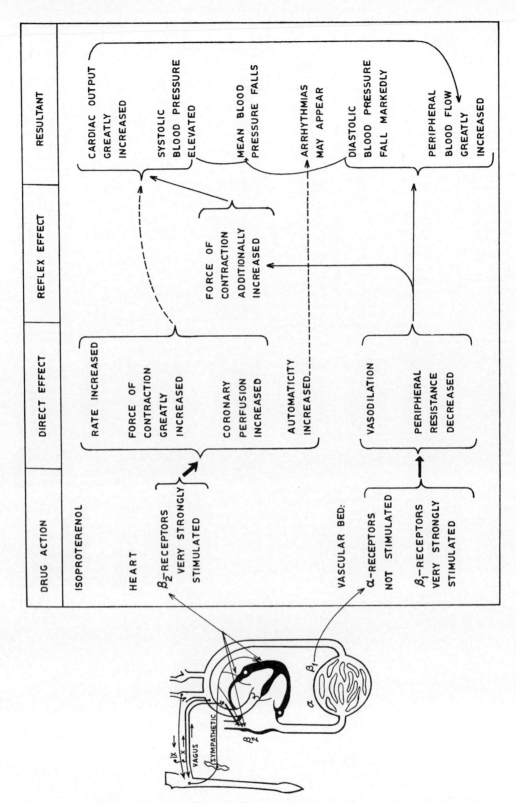

Figure 57. Adapted from Frank H. Netter, M.D., CIBA collection of medical illustrations.

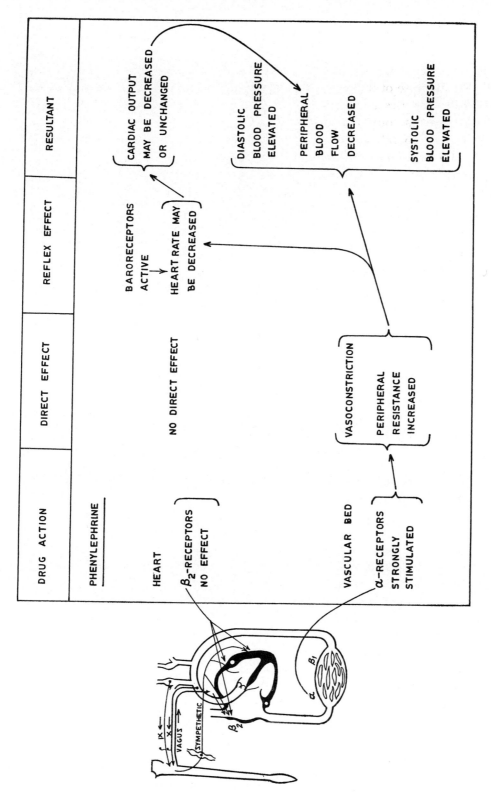

Figure 58. Adapted from Frank H. Netter, M.D., CIBA collection of medical illustrations.

2. Since there is not much rise in mean arterial blood pressure, the baroreceptors are not strongly stimulated.
3. The overall sympathetic tone may not change.
4. Because of the direct, strong, stimulatory effect on the heart, the heart rate increases and tends to overcome any reflex vagal inhibition.
5. Cardiac output is increased.
6. Peripheral blood flow in most areas is increased; but in some areas, such as the skin, it is markedly decreased.

GROUP 2

Isoproterenol

Isoproterenol (Fig. 57) has the following effects:
1. Isoproterenol acts only on beta receptors in the vascular blood and causes a substantial fall in diastolic pressure due to a decrease in total peripheral resistance.
2. Decrease in blood pressure may decrease the baroreceptor activity.
3. Vagal inhibition may be decreased.
4. The marked direct stimulatory effects greatly increase the heart rate.
5. Cardiac output increases and systolic pressure may be maintained.
6. There is marked increase in peripheral blood flow.

GROUP 3

Phenylephrine and Methoxamine

Phenylephrine (Fig. 58) and Methoxamine have the following effects:
1. These drugs have negligible beta receptor activity. They act on alpha receptors in the vascular bed and cause a marked increase in peripheral resistance and hence a marked increase in systolic, diastolic and mean arterial pressure due to peripheral vasoconstriction.
2. Compensatory reflexes arising from the carotid and the aortic arch activate the vagus nerve.
3. The overall sympathetic tone is diminished while there is a marked increase in the vagal tone.
4. Heart rate is decreased.
5. Cardiac output may be decreased.
6. Peripheral blood flow is decreased.
The reflex slowing of the heart may be useful in the treatment of paroxysmal tachycardia.

SECTION THREE

HYPERTENSION

CHAPTER XIII

HYPERTENSION AND TREATMENT

T HE NORMAL ARTERIAL blood pressure in the human being is so variable, it is very difficult to lay down criteria defining when hypertension, or high blood pressure, is present. The difficulty is important when hypertension may exist without exhibiting symptoms. The blood pressure abnormality is discovered only incidentally during a routine examination performed for military, life insurance, or other periodic physical evaluation. Usually when the blood pressure is higher than 140 mm Hg systolic and/or 90 mm Hg diastolic it is considered elevated and abnormal. With a rise in blood pressure, life span may be reduced. Therefore, hypertension should be evaluated fully and, when appropriate, treated.

Several factors (Fig. 59), although not directly involved, may influence the onset and development of hypertension.

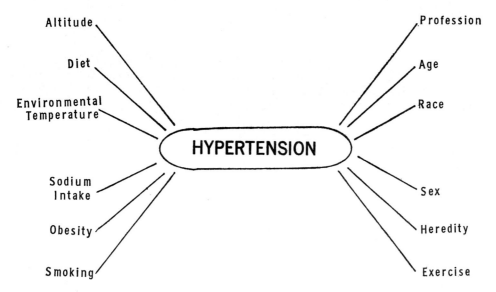

Figure 59. Some of the factors which can influence the onset and rate or development of hypertension.

Profession

Occupation per se, does not play a significant role in the etiology of hypertension. The reaction of the individual to his environment can greatly affect his vascular system, even more than the specific physical or intellectual demands of the individual's job. For example, the executive who has the ability to face major decisions without getting upset may be able to tolerate the vascular effects of stress much better than the person who becomes frustrated by his endless and inconclusive work.

Among hypertensive patients, many are conscientious and perfectionistic, exhibiting high ideals, a strong devotion to duty, and honesty; people who are always dissatisfied with their achievements and are often highly sensitive to criticism.

Age

Hypertension of unknown etiology is less frequent before age 30 and after age 55. Hypertension beginning in the older age group is more likely to be systolic in type and associated with loss of elasticity of the aorta and its main branches.

Race and Sex

Both sex and race seem to play a role in the incidence and severity of hypertensive vascular disease.

American Negroes have a greater incidence of hypertension. It is because the Negro is trained by experience from earliest childhood in the suppression of aggression.

Hypertension appears to be more common in the female than in the male. However, it is better tolerated during the child-bearing years in the female than is hypertension in the male. Following the menopause, the incidence of hypertension in women parallels and may even exceed that in the males.

Heredity

An individual, by reason of inherited traits for hypertension including race and sex, would manifest early in life greater rises in blood pressure in response to environmental stimuli than his counterpart born without these genetic traits.

Exercise

Hypertension may be less frequent and occur at later ages in those who have been more physically active.

Altitude

Hypertension is less common among persons living at high altitudes.

Environmental Temperatures

There is a seasonal influence on blood pressure levels; during summer months blood pressure is slightly lower.

Diet and Salt Intake

The efficacy of a diet low in protein and salt in lowering blood pressure suggests that a high salt intake in diet might be one of the factors responsible for hypertension. This is further supported by the facts that there is; 1) a realtively high incidence of hypertension in areas in which the average consumption of salt is high, and 2) a highly elevated serum sodium content in hypertensive patients.

In contrast to these observations, there are many people who consume excessive amounts of salt and yet do not develop hypertension.

Obesity

It is believed that blood pressure tends to increase with increasing weight, but there is still no definite evidence that obesity per se plays a significant role in the etiology of hypertension. Actually, many very obese patients have low blood pressure and many very lean patient demonstrate severe hypertension.

Smoking

There is enough evidence to conclude that cigarette smoking can contribute to the development of hypertension and other cardiovascular disease. Life expectancy among young men is reduced by an average of 7 to 8 years in heavy (over two packs a day) cigarette smokers and an average of 4 years in light (less than one-half pack a day) cigarette smokers. No substantial evidence has appeared to refute these forecasts.

LABILE HYPERTENSION

Blood pressure may rise initially without any structural pathological changes. Its duration varies depending upon the individual and the surrounding environments. The range is from several months to more than 20 years. During this labile phase there is no evidence of vascular changes and laboratory evaluation will therefore indicate normal organ function. Patients with labile hypertension may not require treatment, but should be watched carefully, since over the course of time such individuals often develop sustained hypertension.

SUSTAINED HYPERTENSION

The simple classification of sustained hypertension is depicted in Figure 60.

Systolic hypertension. It refers to a state in which there is a marked

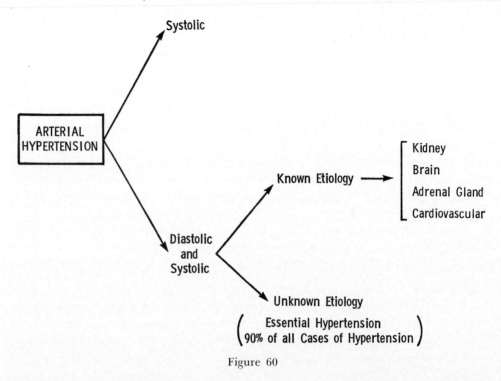

Figure 60

elevation of systolic pressure with little or no elevation of diastolic pressure. In this form of hypertension there is a decreased compliance of the aorta or increased stroke volume (Fig. 61). Decreased compliance is mainly due to arteriosclerosis of the aorta and its main branches. In elderly patients there is high incidence of systolic hypertension with decreased compliance of the aortic wall. This is mainly due to loss of elasticity of the aorta, secondary to arteriosclerosis.

In patients with severe bradycardia, thyrotoxicosis, severe anemia, fever, aortic valvular insufficiency, arteriovenous shunts or fistulas, and the hyperkinetic heart syndrome, systolic hypertension is due to an elevated stroke volume.

Diastolic hypertension. A majority of the hypertensive patients show elevation of diastolic pressure. Diastolic hypertension refers to a state in which there is an increased resistance to the outflow of blood in some portion of the systemic arteriolar bed. Mechanisms responsible for the increase in peripheral resistance and elevation of diastolic pressure are extremely complex.

The many possible mechanisms for the production of high blood pressure are generally grouped into four main classes: endocrine (primarily adrenal glands), renal, cardiovascular, and neural. Several specific diseases in each category are characteristically associated with elevated systemic arterial pressure (Fig. 62).

However, all these causal mechanisms combined will account for the

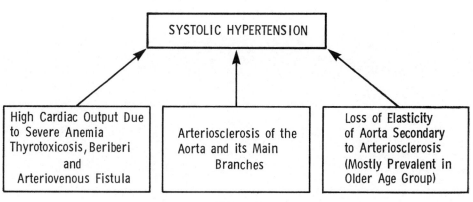

Figure 61

hypertension in only about 5 to 10 percent of all patients. The remaining 90 to 95 percent of these patients have "essential" hypertension.

Essential Hypertension. The term essential hypertension refers to a state of elevated diastolic blood pressure due to increased peripheral resistance for which a specific endocrine or renal basis cannot be found and in which a neural element may be only a mediator of other influences. Thus no specific etiologic factor has been disclosed. This is the meaning of the term essential and its synonym idiopathic, i.e. occurring without cause. Actually, it does not occur without cause; the cause is simply not yet determined. It appears that no single factor is responsible for essential hypertension. It might best be regarded as a multifactorial disease related to abnormalities of the regulatory mechanisms normally concerned with the homeostatic control of arterial pressure. Page has suggested a *mosaic pattern* of how the complex interrelationships of central and sympathetic nervous influences, vascular defects, water and electrolyte metabolism, and cardiac activity can combine to produce the hypertensive state.

Malignant Hypertension. The term malignant hypertension refers to the rapidly progressive phase of hypertensive vascular disease, which may develop *de novo* or may be a sudden change in a previously benign hypertensive course. Manifestations progress rapidly over a period of days to weeks. A small fraction, (1 to 5 percent) of patients with essential hypertension die in this accelerated phase, with severe renal insufficiency and very high levels of arterial pressure. The diastolic pressures reach levels of 140 mm Hg or more. The walls of small arteries and arterioles develop necrosis and concentric collagenous endothelial thickening which results in narrowing of vascular lumen. Examination of the ocular fundi may show papilledema and characteristic hemorrhages, exudates, and advanced vascular narrowing. The lesions of arteriolar necrosis result in cerebral edema, increased intracranial pressure, mental confusion, and seizures.

NEUROGENIC HYPERTENSION

Stress and various acute emotional stimuli raise blood pressure tempo-

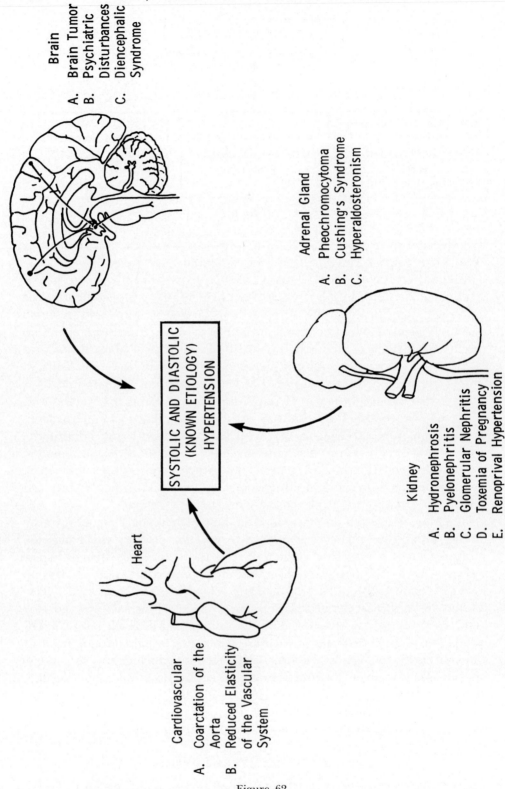

Figure 62

rarily. Such an effect is brought about through neural channels (Fig. 63).
The cortical activity induced by emotional stress affects the cardiovascular
center in the medulla increasing the activity of the heart as well as arteriolar
constriction, especially in great visceral vascular bed. As a result the blood
pressure rises. In addition the adrenal medulla is stimulated causing the
release of epinephrine and norepinephrine which further promotes vaso-

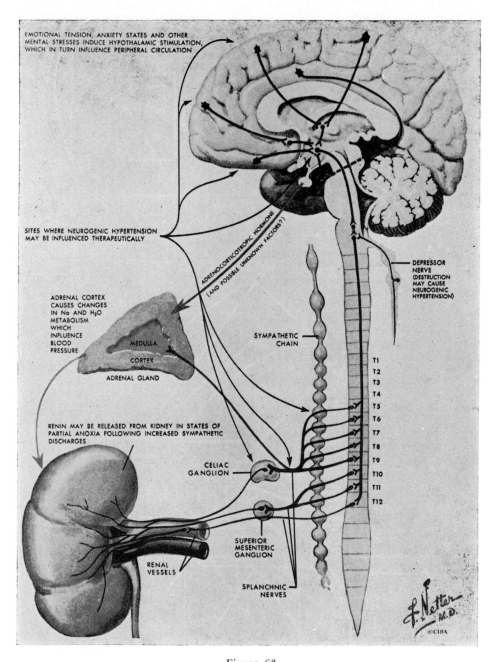

Figure 63

constriction. The blood pressure remains elevated during the emotional storm.

Yet another factor can be brought into play. Simultaneously with the constriction of the peripheral arterioles, there is vasoconstriction of the kidney. Renal vasoconstriction may lead to the release of renin, resulting in the subsequent synthesis of angiotensin. The renin-angiotensin system is a potent stimulator of the adrenal cortex, which in turn releases aldosterone and thereby affecting the electrolytes in the body fluids. This secondary electrolyte effect probably aggravates the hypertensive picture, increasing the transmissibility of impulses at the neuroeffector site of the blood vessel. Certainly an optimal concentration of electrolytes is important to facilitate the transmission of nervous impulses and the ability of norepinephrine to stimulate the blood vessel (Fig. 64). In normal persons the emotional storm is soon over and blood pressure returns to normal. In a compulsive person, these rises would be more frequent, may reach higher levels and tend less and less to return to so called normal values. The walls of the cartoid sinus and aorta begin to stiffen resulting in decreased stimulation of the baroreceptors with the result that their inhibition of vasomotor center diminish and blood pressure is permitted to rise. The continued stress of pressure may finally affect the kidney. The renal circulation may be permanently damaged resulting in excessive amount of release of renin.

The hypothalamus controls the hormonal output of the anterior lobe of the pituitary. Stress may therefore cause the release of adrenocorticotropic

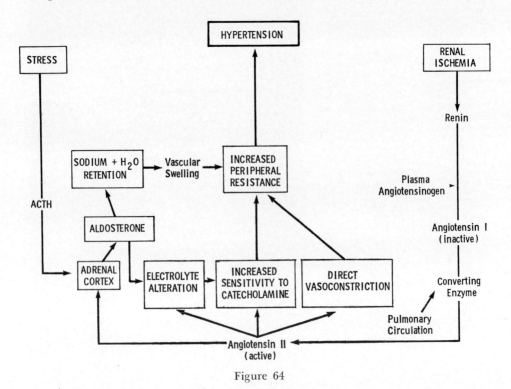

Figure 64

EFFECTS OF ACTH ON ALDOSTERONE PRODUCTION

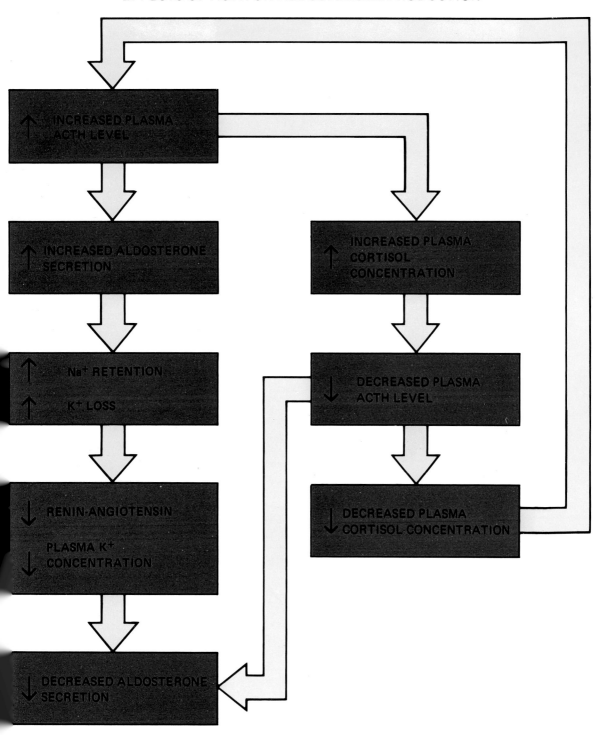

Plate 7 Daily administration of ACTH results in a transient rise in aldosterone secretion. Reprinted with the permission of MEDCOM, Inc. From *Clinician I, The Adrenal Gland,* New York.

PHYSIOLOGICAL AND PATHOLOGICAL FACTORS INFLUENCING THE RENIN–ANGIOTENSIN–ALDOSTERONE SYSTEM

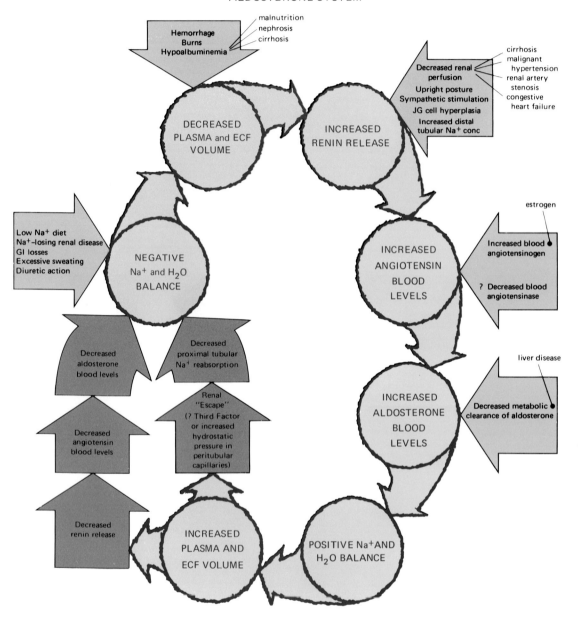

Plate 8 Reprinted with the permission of MEDCOM, Inc. From *Clinician I, The Adrenal Gland,* New York.

IMPORTANCE OF PLASMA RENIN ACTIVITY MEASUREMENTS IN DIAGNOSIS OF PRIMARY ALDOSTERONISM

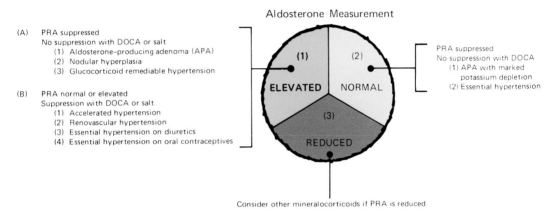

Aldosterone Measurement

(A) PRA suppressed
     No suppression with DOCA or salt
        (1) Aldosterone-producing adenoma (APA)
        (2) Nodular hyperplasia
        (3) Glucocorticoid remediable hypertension

(B) PRA normal or elevated
     Suppression with DOCA or salt
        (1) Accelerated hypertension
        (2) Renovascular hypertension
        (3) Essential hypertension on diuretics
        (4) Essential hypertension on oral contraceptives

(1)   (2)
ELEVATED   NORMAL
(3)
REDUCED

PRA suppressed
No suppression with DOCA
   (1) APA with marked
       potassium depletion
   (2) Essential hypertension

Consider other mineralocorticoids if PRA is reduced

Plate 9 With elevated aldosterone levels (1), renin measurements (A,B) will determine whether the patient has primary or secondary aldosteronism. With low aldosterone levels (3), and reduced PRA, mineralocorticoids other than aldosterone may be responsible for the hypertension. Reprinted with the permission of MEDCOM, Inc. From *Clincian I, The Adrenal Gland,* New York.

hormone (ACTH). ACTH will increase the activity of adrenal cortex to secrete large amounts of aldosterone which may produce hypertension (Fig. 64).

ALDOSTERONISM

Aldosterone is secreted by the zona glomerulus of the adrenal cortex at a rate of 180 to 330 μg/day and is excreted in the urine both as a free aldosterone and as the metabolically inactive degradation tetrahydroaldosterone.

Release of aldosterone is an integral part of the way the body responds to (1) reduced sodium intake, (2) increased potassium intake, (3) exposure to tropical heat, or (4) maintaining an upright posture for prolonged periods of time. Its release is mediated at least through three mechanisms: (1) renin-angiotensin-aldosterone system, (2) changes in plasma potassium concentration, and (3) changes in pituitary corticotropin (ACTH) release (Fig. 64 and Plate 7).

It is believed that oversecretion of aldosterone (hyperaldosteronism) causes hypertension (Fig. 65). (Davis 1970; Biglieri *et al.*, 1972).

There are two types of hyperaldosteronism (Fig. 65):

Primary-aldosteronism resulting from the development of a small tumor in the zona glomerulus of the adrenal cortex which secretes large quantities of aldosterone. The characteristics of primary aldosteronism are presented in Figure 66. In this syndrome the primary defect is in the adrenal cortex.

Primary aldosteronism is one of the more common causes of curable hypertension and should be considered in the evaluation of every case of hypertension. It is commonly relieved by surgical excision of an adrenocortical adenoma.

Secondary aldosteronism results from greater activity in the renin-

Figure 65. *Schematic Representation of Two Varieties of Hyperaldosteronism Involved in Hypertension.*

Hyperaldosteronism can result from (1) renal artery stenosis and, (2) from adrenal cortical adenoma.

In renal artery stenosis either because of a lower blood flow, perfusion pressure or pulse pressure, the kidney sensor on the affected side interprets a lower blood volume. This stimulates the release of renin followed by angiotensin II and aldosterone. This variety of hyperaldosteronism is called secondary, because it is due to excess renin secretion. The defect is in renal sensing element and the increase in blood volume which results from hyperaldosteronism cannot affect the renin secretion.

In functional adrenal cortical adenoma, aldosterone secretion is independent of renin secretion and therefore this type of hyperaldosteronism is called primary. The increased secretion of aldosterone causes increased retention of salt and water, resulting in an increased blood volume which in turn inhibits the secretion of renin. The adrenal tumor is not under the control of the renin mechanism, a decreased level of renin therefore does not affect the secretion of aldosterone by the tumor. Thus the main difference between primary and secondary hyperaldosteronism lies in the finding of a low renin activity in the former and high renin activity in the latter.

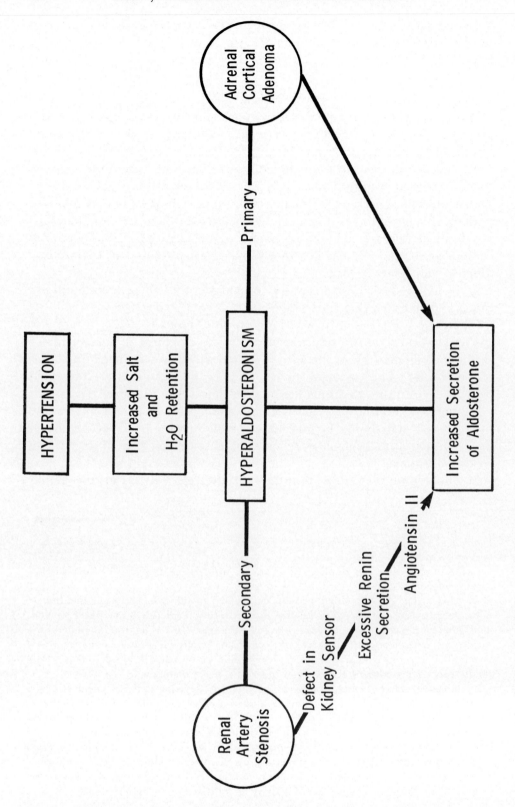

angiotension system. These changes result in increased aldosterone production and release. In this syndrome the defect is not intrinsic to adrenals, but is in the renal sensing elements. (Factors influencing the renin-angiotensin-aldosterone system are presented in Plate 7 and 8).

Aldosterone thus released acts directly upon the distal tubules to bring about the retention of sodium and water in exchange for potassium and hydrogen ions. The consequent sodium retention causes expansion of plasma volume lending to systemic arterial hypertension.

Difference Between Primary and Secondary Hyperaldosteronism

In primary aldosteronism, expansion of plasma volume inhibits the secretion of renin from the juxtaglomerular apparatus. Since the adrenal tumor is not under the control of renin, the secretion of aldosterone from the tumor is not affected. Thus primary aldosteronism is characterized by increased aldosterone secretion in face of low plasma renin. The importance of plasma renin activity measurements in diagnosis of primary aldosteronism is presented in Plate 9.

In secondary aldosteronism, the kidney sensor of the affected side interprets a lower blood volume. This is the signal for specialized cells, the juxtaglomerular cells, to release an enzyme, renin, followed by formation of angiotensin 11 and release of aldosterone. The consequent expansion of plasma volume cannot inhibit the secretion of renin. The defect is in the renal sensing element (Fig. 65).

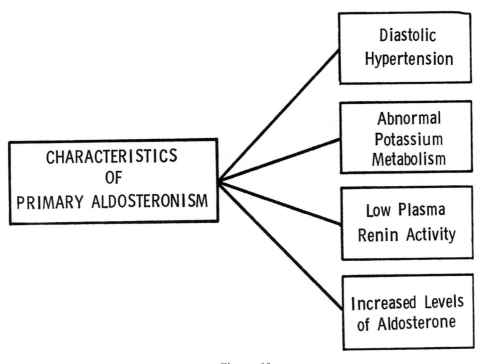

Figure 66

Thus the main difference between primary and secondary hyperaldosteronism lies in the finding of a low renin activity in the former, and of a high renin activity in the latter.

When a person has been standing quietly for four hours, there is a pooling of blood in the lower extremities, causing a transient decrease in cardiac output, renal blood and perfusion of renal afferent arterioles. This, in turn, stimulates renin release. Persons with primary aldosteronism have lower plasma renin activity because of the expanded plasma volume. The decrease in plasma volume which occurs after quiet standing for 4 hours is not sufficient to stimulate renin release; thus renin activity remains low. The difference in renin activity in an upright position differentiates normal persons from patients with primary aldosteronism.

Drugs which cause vasodilation by acting directly on blood vessels, such as sodium nitroprusside or hydralazine, are used to distinguish primary aldosteronism from other hypertension. Since a fall in arterial pressure as a result of administration of these vasodilators stimulates the renin system, the plasma renin activity increases. This response is absent in patients with primary hyperaldosteronism.

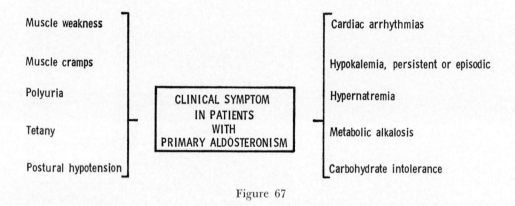

Muscle weakness

Muscle cramps

Polyuria

Tetany

Postural hypotension

CLINICAL SYMPTOM
IN PATIENTS
WITH
PRIMARY ALDOSTERONISM

Cardiac arrhythmias

Hypokalemia, persistent or episodic

Hypernatremia

Metabolic alkalosis

Carbohydrate intolerance

Figure 67

The patients with secondary hyperaldosteronism are responsive to administration of deoxycortico-sterone acetate which readily suppresses the aldosterone levels, whether elevated or normal. This establishes the absence of primary aldosteronism. The clinical symptoms of primary aldosteronism are depicted in Figure 67.

RENIN-ANGIOTENSIN-ALDOSTERONE SYSTEM IN HYPERTENSION INDUCED BY ORAL CONTRACEPTIVE

In some women, oral contraceptives with progestogen-estrogen combinations appear to cause hypertension or to exaggerate their hypertension.

The juxtaglomerular apparatus of the kidney produces increased amounts of renin under the influence of one or both of these hormones. In addition, the liver produces excessive amounts of angiotensinogen. The net result is

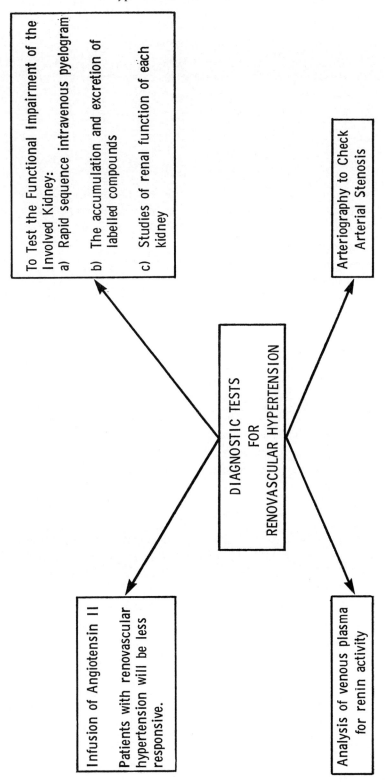

Figure 68

that of greater concentration of angiotensin in the circulation, which, in turn, raises the concentration of aldosterone.

Whether the hypertension results from the elevated levels of plasma angiotensin II, or secondary aldosteronism, or some other effect of these contraceptive agents, is not known at present.

The only rational treatment is withdrawal of the causative agent and its replacement by another type of contraceptive.

RENOVASCULAR HYPERTENSION

Renovascular disease is the most common form of curable hypertension. Lesions such as renal artery stenosis, fibromuscular hyperplasia or renal artery aneurysm which affect the renal blood supply or perfusion pressure may be associated with hypertension.

The most prominent type of lesion (60 percent of all renovascular lesions) is the atheromatous plaque or renal arteriosclerosis. Atheromatous lesions occur mostly in older hypertensive patients (about the age of 60). The plaque affects the proximal one-third of the renal artery. Plaques are also present in association with atherosclerotic lesions in other vessels such as the aorta or other major vessels.

About 20 percent of renal arterial lesions are fibromuscular hyperplasia or fibrous dysplasia of the renal arteries. These lesions are prominent among younger hypertensive patients and are three times more prevalent in females than in males. Fibrous dysplasia of the renal artery occurs most frequently in its distal portion and may involve other arteries and vessels such as the carotid, coronary, celiac, mesenteric and iliac artery. The lesion is characterized by a typical *string of beads* deformity found on angiographic visualization of the renal arteries.

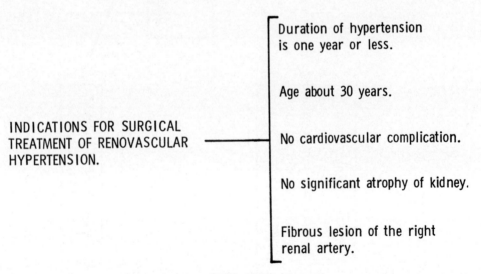

INDICATIONS FOR SURGICAL TREATMENT OF RENOVASCULAR HYPERTENSION.

Duration of hypertension is one year or less.

Age about 30 years.

No cardiovascular complication.

No significant atrophy of kidney.

Fibrous lesion of the right renal artery.

Table XII

There are no suitable diagnostic procedures for renal vascular hypertension; however, several factors should alert the physician to the possible existence of the disease. The diagnosis may be suspected in patients with a history of sudden onset or increased severity of hypertension developing after acute back pain or trauma or with unexplained hypokalemia, and with a negative family history of hypertension. Headaches, congestive heart failure, visual difficulties, anginal pain and nocturia are usually common symptoms in patients with renovascular hypertension. The appropriate diagnostic tests are suggested in Figure 68.

Renovascular hypertension responds like essential hypertension to the usual antihypertensive drugs. Medical treatment is preferred to surgical treatment especially when the risk of operation is high and the prospect for curing the hypertension is not good. The choice of drugs depends upon the severity of the hypertension. Careful follow-up of renal function is necessary if medical treatment is chosen. A rapid-sequence intravenous urogram should be made at least once a year and renal angiography may be repeated once in every two years. The physician can reconsider surgical treatment in case medical treatment fails to control hypertension or if there is progressive atrophy and/or loss of function of affected kidney. Unfortunately, revascularization procedures are not always successful. Nephrectomy

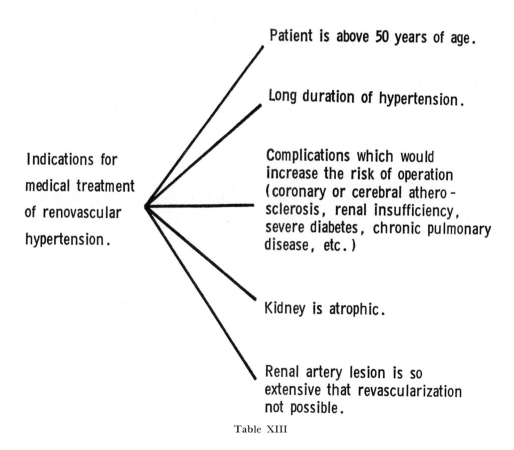

Table XIII

is justified only when the patient is unresponsive to antihypertensive drug and his life is being threatened by hypertension. However, there is evidence to believe that with effective hypotensive treatment, the life expectancy of patients treated with drugs is greater than that of patients surgically treated. Factors favoring medical treatment or surgical treatment are presented in Tables XII and XIII.

THE ROLE OF SYMPATHETIC NERVOUS SYSTEM IN HUMAN HYPERTENSION

The sympathetic nervous system plays a significant role in the pathogenesis of human hypertension. There is increased sympathetic nervous activity in hypertensive diseases of various etiology and the expression of this dysfunction varies with the type and form of hypertension. Except in labile hypertension, there is an increase in peripheral resistance in all forms of human hypertension (Frohlich *et al.*, 1969) Table XIV. Cardiac output may be increased in the early phases of various forms of hypertension (Finkielman *et al.*, 1961; Frohlich *et al.*, 1969) . Increased activity of muscle tone and of basal metabolism was also observed in patients with essential hypertension. The involvement of neurogenic component in the maintenance of elevated blood pressure is also supported by the fact that most drugs used in hypertension interfere in some way with the function of the sympathetic system and that they produce greater falls in blood pressure in hypertensive than in normotensive patients (Green, 1962; Carlsson, 1966; Lucchesi and Whitsitt, 1969; Abrams, 1969) .

Initial studies based on measurement of the urinary excretion of catecholamines and their metabolites in hypertensive patients failed to reveal any consistent alterations in the excretion of norepinephrine, epinephrine,

TABLE XIV

Cardiovascular Alterations in Various Types of Hypertension

Hypertension initially resulting from increased blood volume and/or cardiac output can subsequently become converted to a hypertension from a high peripheral resistance with normal cardiac output.

	Cardiovascular Alterations	
	Cardiac Output	Total Peripheral Resistance
Known Etiology		
Coarctation of Aorta	Increased	Increased
Renal arterial disease	Increased	Increased
Primary aldosteronism	Normal	Increased
Pheochromocytoma	Normal	Increased
Unknown Etiology (Essential)		
Labile	Normal	Normal or Increased
Severe	Decreased	Increased
Essential plus congestive heart failure	Decreased	Increased

vanillylmandelic acid (VMA), and normetanephrine (NMN) in most cases of hypertension, except in pheochromocytoma. In many of these studies, the catecholamines were determined with bioassay methods which lack the sensitivity and specificity of more recent fluorometric methods; and, many of these patients were already on drug therapy or on low sodium diets. Moreover, the impairment of renal function which is likely to influence the pattern of urinary excretion was not evaluated in hypertensive patients since norepinephrine can be significantly reabsorbed by the renal tubule and since norepinephrine excretion can be correlated with urinary flow or volume. Ikoma (1965) has found that the excretion of catecholamines is significantly enhanced in essential hypertensive patients with normal renal function whereas in patients with impaired renal function, urinary excretion of catecholamines is decreased. When measurements were made under more standardized conditions, in unmedicated hypertensive patients, with normal renal function, it was found that urinary levels of norepinephrine, VMA, or NMN were significantly elevated. A highly significant correlation was found between the systolic or diastolic blood pressure and the urinary excretion of norepinephrine in the normotensive and hypertensive patients (Ikoma, 1965; Nestel and Doyle, 1968). When patients are given drug treatment, the blood pressure is lowered and there is concomitant reduction of urinary excretion of norepinephrine. This correlation between blood pressure and urinary catecholamines in humans is consistent with the inverse relationship found between the turnover and storage of norepinephrine and the systolic blood pressure in DOCA-hypertensive rats and in rats subjected to a low sodium diet (de Champlain *et al;* 1972).

Thus it appears that there is increased secretion of catecholamine in hypertensive patients. This is further supported by the fact that the sympathetic response to mental stress or to tilting caused a greater increase in the excretion of norepinephrine in hypertensive patients than in normotensive subjects (Nestel, 1969; Nestel and Esler, 1970).

Since plasma catecholamines are very low, precise measurement of changes in catecholamines is very difficult. Plasma catecholamine levels in hypertensive patients were found either normal (Hoobler *et al.*, 1954; Manger, 1962) or increased (Hirano *et al.*, 1969). More recently, Engleman and coworkers (1970), using a highly sensitive double isotope technique, reported that circulating catecholamine levels in essential hypertension subjects were about twice those of normotensive subjects.

Gitlow and coworkers (1964) found that in patients with essential hypertension tritiated norepinephrine declines more rapidly in their plasma after intravenous infusion suggesting impairment in the storage and binding of norepinephrine in adrenergic terminals. In subsequent studies, Gitlow and coworkers (1969) injected ^{3}H-norepinephrine and measured the amount of ^{3}H-norepinephrine and metabolites excreted in the urine during the following 24 hours. They found the urinary excretion of catecholamines significantly greater in hypertensive patients, indicating that the turnover rate of epinephrine is probably increased in the vascular sympathetic fibers. The abnormality in the pattern of excretion of tritiated norepinephrine and metabolites in hypertensive patients is strikingly similar to the pattern of urinary excretion in DOCA-hypertensive rats (Fig. 69) after an identical treatment (Krakoff, *et al.,* 1967).

Since patients with essential hypertension do not constitute a homogenous population of patients, the sympathetic system therefore may play a variable role in the pathogenesis and maintenance of hypertension. In some of these hypertensive patients, there is increased activity of the sympathetic nervous system. In other patients with normal sympathetic activity and normal norepinephrine metabolism, there is increased sensitivity of the adrenergic receptors to normal amounts of the neurotransmitter. Changes in catecholamine metabolism may be a primary factor in some patients, while in others such changes may be secondary to hemodynamic disturbances or to circulating substances such as angiotensin. Furthermore, the evaluation time is critical since the sympathetic nervous system may be responsible for only one stage of the disease. Arteriosclerosis and renal disease, which develop in the course of chronic hypertension, may modify considerably the activity of the sympathetic system. Thus the factors and mechanisms responsible for the maintenance of hypertension may change even during its evolution. However, it is difficult at present to determine whether the sympathtic nervous system plays a primary role in the pathogenesis of certain forms of hypertension or whether it contributes only to certain stages of the hypertensive disease. It is likely that both possibilities exist in human and experimental hypertension. Alteration in turnover rate of norepinephrine may precede the rise in blood pressure in certain cases, whereas in renal hypertension, the sympathetic nervous system becomes prominent only in the chronic stage.

Although hypertension may be initiated by different etiological factors, it is possible that many of these factors increase the blood pressure indirectly by influencing the activity of the sympathetic system. The sympathetic nervous system would then serve as a common pathway for different etiological factors. (Fig. 69A)

EFFECTS OF HYPERTENSION

When high blood pressure persists for a prolonged period of time, clinical manifestations reflecting the underlying pathological sequele of the hypertensive state usually became apparent. Initially they include headache, dizziness, nose bleeding and breathlessness on exertion. At a later stage, the main complications arise from the secondary effects of hypertension on the retina (Fig. 70), the brain (Fig. 71), the heart (Fig. 72) and kidney (Fig. 73). If unaltered by therapy they often ultimately result in illness and death.

CONTROL OF CIRCUMSTANCES

Myocardial infarctions and cerebral vascular accidents occur somewhat

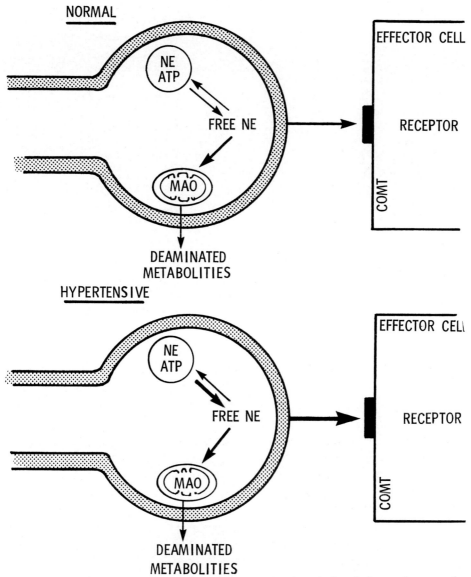

Figure 69. Diagrammatic representation of the alterations induced due to hypertension in the storage and metabolism of norepinephrine.

Under normal conditions norepinephrine is bound within dense core vesicle, presumably to ATP and protein to form a stable complex. Norepinephrine which is not bound is released into the cytoplasm. Norepinephrine which is released into the cytoplasm is mostly exposed to the action of monoamine oxidase. Norepinephrine which is released into the synaptic cleft is partly exposed to catechol-o-methyl transferase, while another part is taken up by the nerves and bound again into the granules and the remainder diffuses away from the site of liberation. A very small amount exerts its action on receptors. In the hypertensive animals more norepinephrine appears to be released from the storage vesicle. This results in lower endogenous levels of norepinephrine in the tissue and in the increased excretion of norepinephrine and the deaminated and O-methylated metabolites in the kidney and urine.

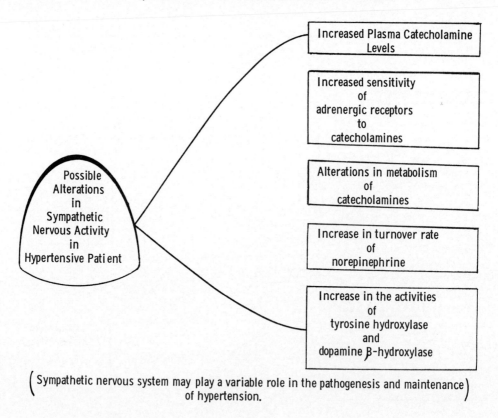

Possible
Alterations
in
Sympathetic
Nervous Activity
in
Hypertensive Patient

Increased Plasma Catecholamine
Levels

Increased sensitivity
of
adrenergic receptors
to
catecholamines

Alterations in metabolism
of
catecholamines

Increase in turnover rate
of
norepinephrine

Increase in the activities
of
tyrosine hydroxylase
and
dopamine β-hydroxylase

(Sympathetic nervous system may play a variable role in the pathogenesis and maintenance)
of hypertension.

more frequently among patients with labile hypertension than among those with fixed hypertension. These findings suggest the need for individual attention to the control of circumstances that may cause the blood pressure to fluctuate dangerously. It is necessary to reduce environmental stress in treating these patients. Maintenance of adequate therapy is also important to inhibit a sudden increase in blood pressure, which may follow even a brief discontinuance of medication or the development of tolerance and resistance to further therapy as a result of suboptimal dosage.

PROGRAM OF TREATMENT

The attitude of physicians towards hypertension differs. Some think that drugs should not be given to treat it. Most authorities, however, recommend that anyone under 65 years of age whose diastolic pressure is more than 100 mm Hg. should receive drug therapy to lower the blood pressure. Men under 45 years of age, women under 35 years of age, and Negroes of either sex at any age whose diastolic pressure is more than 90 mm Hg. should also be treated with drugs to control the blood pressure.

Statistical evidence indicates that in hypertensive patients, control of blood pressure does reduce morbidity and improves the prognosis. Survival rate is proportional to the extent of blood pressure reduction by drugs and

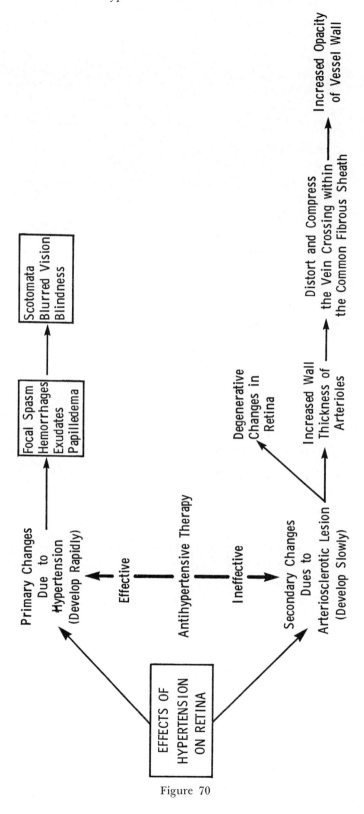

Figure 70

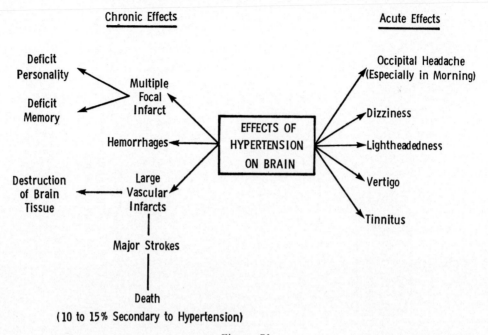

Figure 71

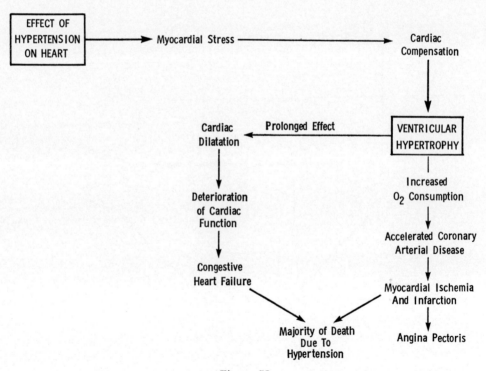

Figure 72

to the kidney function at the beginning of therapy. Thus, early identification and treatment may lessen incidences of strokes and prolong life. A list of routine laboratory tests is given in Figure 74.

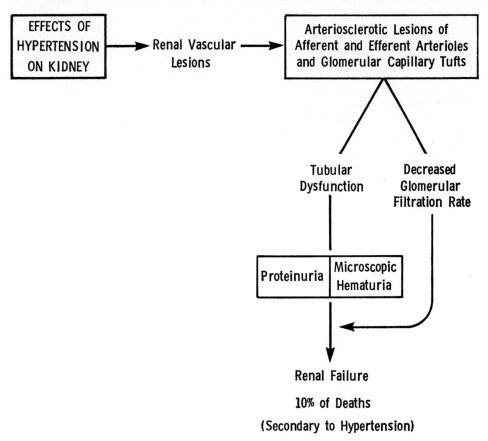

Figure 73

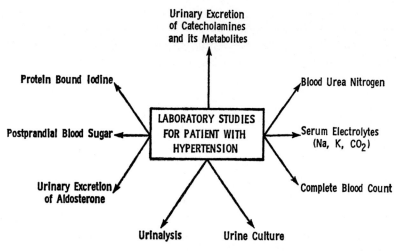

Figure 74

Antihypertensive therapy virtually has eliminated heart failure as a cause of death. The most frequent causes of death in treated hypertensive patients are associated vascular disease and renal failure.

In order to determine whether or not the hypertension is secondary and the cause reversible, a complete inventory of the patient's health is necessary (Table 15). If the cause is reversible, therapy should be outlined in detail and directed at the cause. Some of the known factors adversely affecting the prognosis in hypertensive patients are presented in Figure 75.

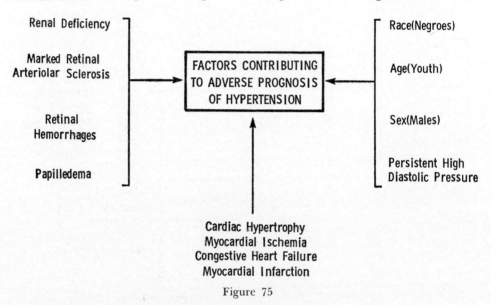

Figure 75

That treatment should be carried out patiently and rigorously should be impressed upon the patient. It should also include:

1. *Weight control.* In all forms of cardiovascular disease, obesity is to be avoided. Fat adds useless extra weight which has to be carried at the cost of an additional energy output by an already overworked heart. Hypertension increases the workload of the heart, which is further enhanced by larger amounts of adipose tissue requiring greater circulation. Particularly in cases of mild hypertension, a reduction of weight to a figure below that regarded as normal for individuals of the sex, age and height of the patient may have a more valuable therapeutic effect than any form of drug treatment. It is therefore necessary that the patient should try to maintain his proper weight.

2. *Mental and physical rest* are also extremely important. All anxiety states should be vigorously treated to effect good results.

3. The *diet* must be well balanced and it should not include excessive amounts of proteins. Water should be freely permitted but sodium intake should be restricted. A strict restriction in sodium intake reduces the blood pressure in hypertension. Dietetic methods are undoubtedly effective but irksome to patients and are rarely employed now. It is doubtful

TABLE XV
Work Sheet for Study of Hypertensive Patient

Routine Studies	
History and physical exam	Routine studies may indicate etiology of the hypertension
Funduscopic evaluation	
Complete blood count	
Urinalysis	Necessary for the evaluation of severity and progress of
Blood urea nitrogen	the disease, results of therapy, and prognosis
Chest roentgenogram or orthodiagram	
Electrocardiogram	
Intravenous pyelogram	
Special Diagnostic Studies	
Urine Culture	Asymptomatic pyelonephritis may be cause of hypertension
Catecholamines (blood, urine) Vanillylmandelic Acid (VMA— urine)	Chemical tests—best screening tests for pheochromocytoma
Regitine test	Pharmacologic tests may be performed jointly with chemi-
Histamine test	cal test to increase accuracy of diagnosis
Tyramine test	
Renal arteriogram; perirenal CO_2 study	To localize pheochromocytoma
Electrolytes Na, K, CO_2 (blood)	May indicate aldosteronism (primary or secondary)
Electrolytes (urine)	Often abnormal secondary to thiazide therapy
Aldosterone (urine)	
Renal arteriogram	Diagnosis of renovascular hypertension
Differential renal function	Diagnosis of branch renal artery lesion; helpful in bilateral renal artery stenosis
Radioactive renogram	Possible value as screening tests for renovascular hyper-
Scanning tests	tension, but not definitive
Renal biopsy	Occult pyelonephritis, juxtaglomerular granularity, histo- logic evidence of prognostic significance
Renin in peripheral venous blood	Separate primary from secondary hyperaldosteronism
Differential renal venous renin or angiotensin	Determine functional nature of anatomic renal artery stenosis

Reprinted through courtesy of Lea & Febiger from Seller *et al.: Cardiac and Vascular Diseases,* (Vol. II)

whether a moderate restriction of salt intake influences blood pressure. "It is not the sodium as an ion, but salt as a volume holder that is most important in the hypertensive effect." Low sodium diet is unnecessary when thiazide diuretics are being used.

4. *General hygienic measures* such as laxatives, vacations, rest in bed after meals, plenty of sleep, and prompt care of infections are to be urged.

5. *Frequent visits to the physician* are necessary for follow-up and, most important, to keep the patient on his medical regimen and the reminder that his illness requires continual treatment. A major reason for poor control of blood pressure is failure to continue medication.

6. *Prevention* of cardiac damage is accomplished by proper treatment of hypertension. The treatment of complications is instituted only after attempted prevention has failed or if they exist at the initial examination.

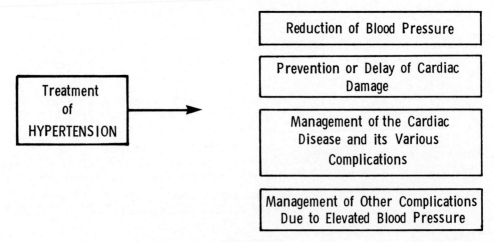

Figure 76

7. *Cigarette smoking* enhances the mortality rate of the hypertensive patients and, therefore, the patient should be encouraged to quit smoking. If the patient finds it a severely distressing experience, the anxiety and upset due to abstention from smoking may exceed the benefits derived therefrom. Under such circumstances it is wise not to require this.

The aim of therapy (Fig. 76) is to lower the diastolic pressure to as normal as possible. A reduction in blood pressure usually relieves the reversible secondary manifestations. The extent of relief does not depend on the method employed to lower the blood pressure, but on how effectively and consistently it has been reduced.

To reduce the elevated blood pressure it is logical to accomplish this through the mechanism responsible for the normal regulation of blood pressure. These are:

1. Cardiac output
2. Volume of the blood
3. Viscosity of the blood
4. Peripheral resistance
5. Vascular capacity

However, all these factors are normal in hypertensive subjects except peripheral resistance which is increased.

CHOICE OF DRUG

An ideal hypotensive drug will be one that provides the most effective blood pressure control with the least side effects. Some of the desirable properties of a hypotensive drug are given in Figure 77.

In recent years, adjusting the treatment to the requirements of each patient has been emphasized. Obviously, as new drugs with different characteristics become available, the choice of medication grows more difficult. The planning of a suitable regimen is now a problem of some complexity, since hypertensive patients have great variation in responsiveness to indi-

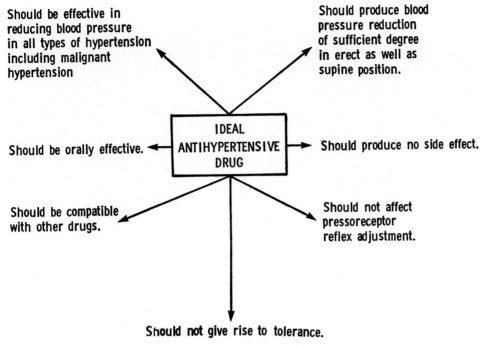

Should be effective in reducing blood pressure in all types of hypertension including malignant hypertension

Should produce blood pressure reduction of sufficient degree in erect as well as supine position.

Should be orally effective.

IDEAL ANTIHYPERTENSIVE DRUG

Should produce no side effect.

Should be compatible with other drugs.

Should not affect pressoreceptor reflex adjustment.

Should not give rise to tolerance.

Figure 77

vidual drugs. Therefore, it is always advisable to test a variety of regimens before settling on one.

The success of the therapeutic regimen selected often depends on the precision with which the dosage of each drug is adjusted in accordance with the patient's response at progressive stages of treatment.

Antihypertensive drugs are usually given in combinations since it provides a number of advantages to the clinician. The same antihypertensive effect may be achieved using smaller doses of the individual drugs. This reduces the incidence of severity of adverse reactions and delays the development of tolerance. Sometimes, when the adverse or side effects of one drug are particularly undesirable, for example reduction in renal blood flow caused by ganglionic blocking agents, the additional use of a drug having an opposite side effect, (e.g. hydralazine) may be beneficial.

Most of the drugs used to treat hypertension lower arterial blood pressure primarily by depressing the sympathetic nervous system and thereby decreasing peripheral vascular resistance. These drugs cause sympathetic blockade by acting on different anatomical sites (Fig. 78). Such drugs may act centrally, may depress transmission in sympathetic nerves anywhere along the afferent or reflex pathway involved in blood pressure regulation, and/or may interfere with sympathetic control or arteriolar tone by inhibiting transmission in the adrenergic neuron or in the sympathetic ganglion.

In addition, the diuretics, (especially thiazide diuretics), which act primarily on electrolytes at the neuroeffector site are being used for treatment

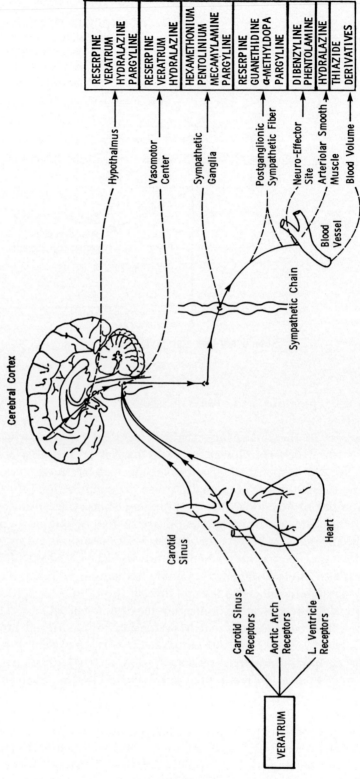

Figure 78

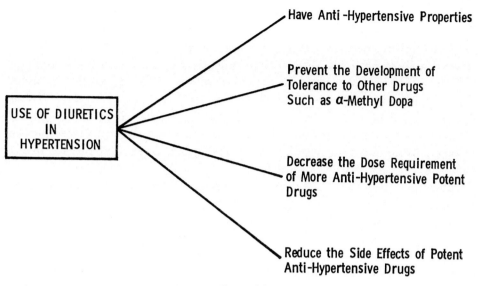

Figure 79

of hypertension (Fig. 79). These thiazide diuretics are not particularly potent as antihypertensive agents in their own right, but they potentiate the action of the sympathetic nervous system depressants, reducing the dosage requirement of the latter and consequently the side effects.

The diuretic drugs are used in a fixed dose equivalent to about 500 mg of chlorothiazide (Diuril®) twice daily, or 1000 mg per day. The dose can be somewhat larger initially, beginning with 1000 mg twice a day and subsequently reducing this after 4 days to 500 mg twice a day, or the equivalent of other diuretic agents. If these alone are insufficient, the sympathetic blocking drugs may be used in addition.

In treating the patient who develops hypokalemia, spironolactone or triamterene should be administered. This will antagonize the potassium loss and will enhance the natriuretic effect. If the patient has a tendency to loose large amounts of potassium, this treatment is preferable to giving a large amount of potassium in the diet each day. Once the patient is adjusted, intake of potassium is regulated to maintain a normal level.

The choice of a sympathetic blocking drug depends on diastolic pressure levels. When the diastolic pressure is less than 100 mm Hg. (mild hypertension) rauwolfia alkaloid should be tried. When it is less than 130 mm Hg. i.e. moderate hypertension, it is appropriate to try α-methyldopa (Aldomet) in a dose of 250 mg a day which is increased by 250 mg each week to as much as 1500 or 2000 mg a day until the diastolic blood pressure is not over 100 mm of mercury when taken with the patient standing. Patients who do not respond adequately to α-methyldopa should be tried on guanethidine.

When the diastolic pressure is over 130 mm Hg., hypertension is considered severe and there are usually changes in the optic fundi, cardiac or renal decompensation or rapid progression of cardiac or renal damage. It is better to start with guanethidine, or ganglionic blocking agents; some include pargyline in this latter group. Among the last three, guanethidine is undoubtedly prominent. The initial daily dose of guanethidine should be 12.5 mg; this is increased at weekly intervals by 12.5 mg until the blood pressure is reduced below 150/100 when the patient is standing. If the orthostatic effect of the guanethidine plus diuretics alone is too great, methyldopa may be added to the regimen and the dosage of guanethidine reduced. With the proper adjustment of dosages between these two drugs the desired effect can be obtained.

Pargyline (Eutonyl) is nearly as potent as guanethidine when used in combination with a diuretic agent. However, the primary indication for its use is to treat those patients who, for one reason or another, cannot tolerate guanethidine and/or methyldopa, or do not respond adequately to these drugs, or who have associated psychic depression. Since it is a monoamine oxidase inhibitor, pargyline will usually alleviate psychic depression at the same time that it reduces blood pressure. This is another indication for using the drug.

In the treatment of the patient who has advanced renal damage from severe hypertension, an attempt should be made to arrest the progressive renal damage resulting from the blood pressure elevation without actually reducing the glomerular filtration rate which occurs as a result of the blood pressure reduction. Methyldopa is remarkably effective in this regard. Methyldopa maintains cardiac output while peripheral vascular resistance is reduced. Thereby, renal blood flow is maintained despite the blood pressure reduction; consequently, there is minimal depression of the glomerular filtration rate and renal excretory function.

One of the major problems, particularly during the first few months of antihypertensive therapy, is the development of tolerance of drugs. Progressively increasing doses of drugs are required to control blood pressure effectively.

HYPERTENSIVE EMERGENCIES

When a patient's life is threatened as a direct consequence of an acute elevation in blood pressure, a "hypertensive" emergency may be said to exist. Rapid lowering of blood pressure even at the risk of inducing side effects may be life-saving. It requires parenteral administration of antihypertensive drugs. These emergencies include:

1. Hypertensive encephalopathy
2. Acute left ventricular failure
3. Intractable angina or coronary insufficiency: Lowering of the blood pressure may decrease cardiac work and relieve anginal pain. The blood pressure should be lowered cautiously. During the acute stage of myocardial infarction or coronary insufficiency, usually no attempt is made to lower the elevated blood pressure.
4. Malignant hypertension

5. Toxemia of pregnancy
6. Acute glomerular nephritis
7. Severe hypertension in postoperative stages
8. Pressor episode due to pheochromocytoma

The patient should be put in a quiet ward where extensive nursing aid is available, and close observation is possible. Anti-convulsant precautions should be observed including side rails for the bed and a handy tongue depressor.

The drug of choice for the management of acute hypertensive emergencies is parenteral reserpine. If reserpine alone is ineffective, short-acting ganglionic blocking agents, preferably trimethaphan, are used, because they have a rapid onset of action. They are administered intramuscularly or by continuous intravenous drip. The patient must be observed carefully for occurrence of hypotension or its consequence. If the situation arises, pressor agents may be used to raise the blood pressure.

Elevation of blood pressure due to pheochromocytoma can be rapidly controlled by adrenergic blocking drugs such as phenoxybenzamine. It is usually given intravenously.

When the blood pressure has been brought under control, efforts should be directed to correct the underlying cause of the hypertensive episode. In case it is difficult, a long term therapy should be planned.

CHAPTER XIV

PHEOCHROMOCYTOMA

THE ADRENAL GLAND in man contains the physiologically and embryologically distinct cortex and medulla within one capsule. The cortex originates from the mesonephric blastema and is mesodermal in origin, whereas the adrenal medulla originates from the neural crest and is ectodermal in origin. The adrenal medulla arises in common with the sympathetic chain, the ganglia, and the celiac plexus.

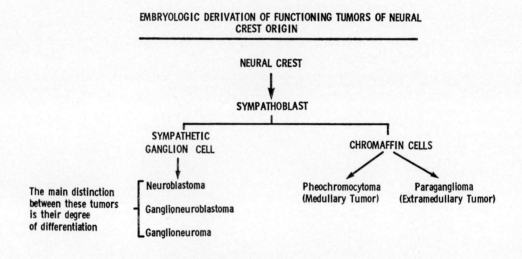

EMBRYOLOGIC DERIVATION OF FUNCTIONING TUMORS OF NEURAL CREST ORIGIN

NEURAL CREST

SYMPATHOBLAST

SYMPATHETIC GANGLION CELL

CHROMAFFIN CELLS

The main distinction between these tumors is their degree of differentiation

Neuroblastoma

Ganglioneuroblastoma

Ganglioneuroma

Pheochromocytoma (Medullary Tumor)

Paraganglioma (Extramedullary Tumor)

All tumors may secrete catecholamines and produce hypertension and metabolic disorders.

Figure 80

At an early stage of embryonic development, primordial adrenergic cells (neuroblasts) begin to differentiate either into sympathetic ganglion cells or into chromaffin cells. Some of the chromaffin cells have an additional capacity to synthesize epinephrine from norepinephrine. As the embryo develops, chromaffin cells come to lie in a number of clusters throughout the retroperitoneal region, the largest of which are the adrenal medullae and the Organs of Zuckerkandl (located on either side of the aorta near the origin of the inferior mesenteric artery). Small groups of chromaffin cells also adhere to each sympathetic ganglion and thus are known as paraganglia.

Tumors of chromaffin tissue are of two types, the pheochromocytoma and the paraganglioma (Fig. 80). This latter term usually applies to chromaffin tumors of neural crest origin beyond the confines of the adrenal gland.

The ganglion or nonchromaffin cells include the neuroblastoma, the ganglioneuroblastoma, and the ganglioneuroma. The only distinction between these two tumors is their degree of differentiation. All tumors arising from the cells of neural crest origin may secrete catecholamines and produce hypertension. Recognition of the endocrine nature of these tumors rests on the urinary measurement of norepinephrine, epinephrine, and their metabolites (metanephrine and vanillylmandelic acid) in the blood or urine, or following excision, measurement of the catecholamine in the tumor.

Most symptoms and signs associated with pheochromocytoma are due entirely to the effect of circulating catecholamines secreted by the tumor. The patient history supports this since (1) catecholamines levels are elevated both in blood and urine during attack and (2) manifestation of pheochromocytoma are antagonized by α-blocking drugs such as phenoxybenzamine and phentolamine. However, misdiagnosis is common, because the symptoms may also mimic those of more common disorders such as thyrotoxicosis, anxiety, diabetes mellitus or hyperventilation (Melmon, 1968).

The symptoms of a pheochromocytoma are extremely variable (Fig. 81). The variability in symptom is based on whether the release of catecholamine from tumors is constant or intermittant. These patients are hypertensive all or most of the time; few patients are intermittantly hypertensive during attacks which may last anywhere from a few minutes to a few hours. Orthostatic hypotension is most common in these patients. This is one of the important diagnostic features of pheochromocytoma, since in most other untreated hypertensive patients blood pressure measured during standing is equal to or greater than that during the supine position.

DIAGNOSIS

The most important diagnostic test for pheochromocytoma is to determine free catecholamines or metabolies in a 24-hour urine sample (Fig. 82). These values are elevated in 90 to 95 percent of patients. Persons taking tetracycline, quinidine, α-methyl dopa, isoproterenol, monoamine oxidase inhibitors, barbiturates, thiazides, reserpine, hydralazine, guanethidine, ganglionic blocking agents, cardiac glycosides, or phentolamine, may yield erroneous values. If possible, treatment may be discontinued for a day or two for collection of the urine specimen. Careful correlation between a patient's clinical condition and the laboratory findings should be made.

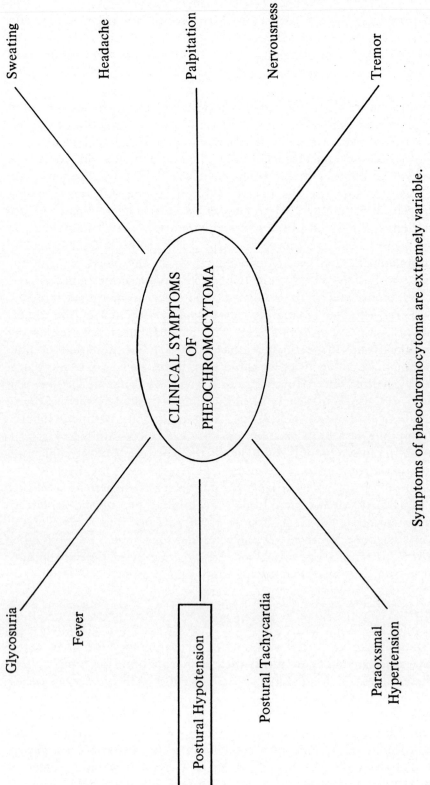

Sweating

Headache

Palpitation

Nervousness

Tremor

CLINICAL SYMPTOMS
OF
PHEOCHROMOCYTOMA

Glycosuria

Fever

Postural Hypotension

Postural Tachycardia

Paraoxsmal
Hypertension

Symptoms of pheochromocytoma are extremely variable.

Figure 81

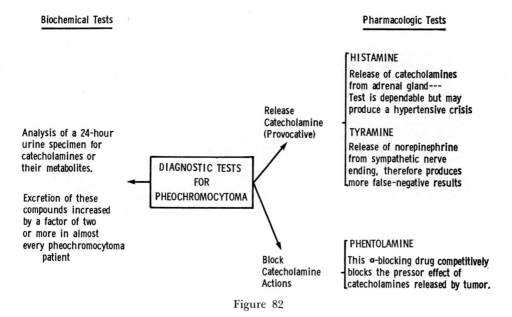

Figure 82

The test should be repeated in patients who are borderline. A persistant increase in values is strongly suggestive of pheochromocytoma.

A rather common diagnostic problem is the patient who gives a history of attacks suggestive of pheochromocytoma, and yet who has a normal excretion of catecholamines and metabolites.

The crucial diagnostic test under these circumstances is the determination of free urinary norepinephrine and epinephrine in a carefully timed urine specimen which brackets the attack (Crout, 1966). The demonstration of a normal excretion of norepinephrine and epinephrine during a period of hypertension excludes pheochromocytoma as the cause of the hypertension.

Pharmacological Test

The drugs used in the diagnosis of pheochromocytoma are of two types: *provocative* drugs, such as histamine, tyramine or glucagon which release catecholamines from increased stores, and *blocking* drugs such as phentolamine (α-adrenergic blocking drug) which blocks the action of circulating catecholamines and thereby causes a fall in blood pressure.

Both of these tests can cause a false positive, or false negative response. Therefore, pharmacologic tests should be supplemented with adequate chemical tests (Fig. 82).

TREATMENT

The ultimate treatment consists of surgical removal of the tumor. Removal of tumor leads to cure if the operation is performed prior to the occurrance of permanent damage to the kidney or to other organs. Surgical operation poses two serious problems:

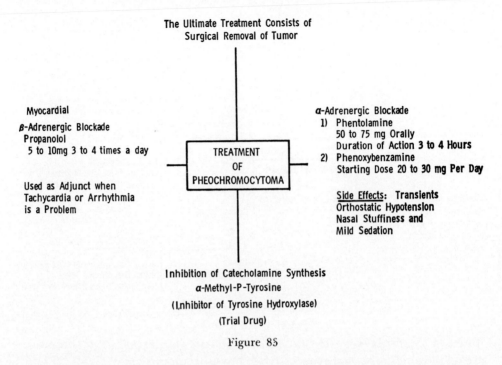

The Ultimate Treatment Consists of
Surgical Removal of Tumor

Myocardial

β-Adrenergic Blockade
Propanolol
  5 to 10mg 3 to 4 times a day

Used as Adjunct when
Tachycardia or Arrhythmia
is a Problem

TREATMENT
OF
PHEOCHROMOCYTOMA

α-Adrenergic Blockade
1) Phentolamine
   50 to 75 mg Orally
   Duration of Action **3 to 4 Hours**
2) Phenoxybenzamine
   Starting Dose 20 to **30 mg Per Day**

Side Effects: **Transients**
Orthostatic Hypotension
Nasal Stuffiness and
Mild Sedation

Inhibition of Catecholamine Synthesis
α-Methyl-P-Tyrosine
(Inhibitor of Tyrosine Hydroxylase)
(Trial Drug)

Figure 85

1. RELEASE OF CATECHOLAMINES DURING EITHER ANESTHESIA OR MANIPU-LATION OF TUMOR: It is necessary that surgical procedure is preceded by therapy with α-adrenergic blocking drugs such as phenoxybenzamine or phentolamine. Phentolamine is preferred since it does not cause release of catecholamines. It is usually administered orally 50 mg every four to six hours for four to six days prior to the operation. Cyclopropane anesthesia is contraindicated since it sensitizes the myocardium to the action of pressor amines and therefore may lead to cardiac arrhythmia. If the situation warrants, the blood vessel to the tumor should be ligated prior to manipulation of the tumor. At the time of surgery, phentolamine can control hypertension.

2. HYPOTENSION AFTER SURGERY: This may be controlled by the infusion of norepinephrine. In cases of malignant pheochromocytoma or in benign tumors, long-term management is accomplished with oral α-adrenergic blocking drug or drugs (Fig. 83) that prevent the synthesis of catechol-amines (Engleman and Sjoerdsma, 1971). Most patients with untreated pheochromocytoma die of cardiovascular disease rather than their tumor per se. Blockade of cardiovascular and metabolic effects of circulating catecholamines with adrenergic blocking drugs may improve in the survivals of many years (Engelman and Sjoerdsma, 1964). Brunjes *et al;* (1960) reported that patients have usually low blood volume and, in particular, a greatly reduced red cell mass. This may be cured preoperatively by transfusion with packed red cells (Johns and Brunjes, 1962).

CHAPTER XV

PHARMACOLOGY OF ANTIHYPERTENSIVE AGENTS

THE DRUGS MOST commonly used alone or in combination for treatment of the vast majority of patients with hypertension are:
1. Ganglionic blocking agents
2. Reserpine
3. Alpha-methyldopa
4. Guanethidine
5. MAO inhibitors
6. Thiazide (Diuretics)
7. Hydralazine

GANGLIONIC BLOCKING AGENT

The most potent antihypertensive drugs are those which block the ganglionic transmission through the ganglion without causing depolarization. They are called ganglionic blocking agents.

They compete for the receptors on which acetylcholine acts, and the acetylcholine released from the nerve terminals of preganglionic fibers is ineffective in stimulating the ganglion cells which it can no longer depolarize.

With these drugs, it is possible to control high blood pressure and to reverse the eye changes, retinal hemorrhages and papilloedema.

The ganglion blockers tend to produce little or no fall in arterial pressure when the patient is supine, and a small, moderate or large fall when the patient stands, which is due to a fall in cardiac output and a failure of reflex vasoconstriction. It is usual, therefore, to have the patient out of bed as much as possible, and when in bed, to have his head and shoulders raised.

These agents produce unpleasant symptoms by blocking parasympathetic ganglia as well as sympathetic ganglia.

Even moderate doses may produce impairment of visual accommodation, dryness of the mouth, nausea, constipation, paralytic ileus, failure of erection and ejaculation, retention of urine and other side effects which have led to their discontinuance in the long-term treatment of hypertension. After each injection, there is a period of postural hypotension, which still remains a drawback of all the more recently introduced agents, with the exception of α-methyldopa, etc.

These drugs have been replaced by adrenergic neuron blocking drugs which only block the sympathetic component of the autonomic nervous system and therefore have no side effects of parasympathetic blockade.

Comparison of ganglionic blockade with selective sympathetic inhibition is presented in Table XVI.

Ganglionic blocking agents are useful in a hypertensive emergency because they have a rapid onset of action. Short-acting ganglionic blocking agents are used in the treatment of severe hypertension associated with acute left ventricular failure. They are administered intramuscularly or by continuous intravenous drip.

The patient must be observed carefully for the occurrence of hypotension or its consequences. If the situation warrants, a pressor agent may be used to raise the blood pressure.

Hexamethonium and pentolinium continue to be extremely useful drugs for intravenous injection in left ventricular failure and hypertensive fits.

The ganglionic blocking agents are used only when patients with severe hypertension on thiazide, reserpine and/or hydralazine therapy have failed to respond to the addition of guanethidine or α-methyldopa.

The commonly used blocking agents are mecamylamine, chlorisondamine, and pentolinium tartrate.

The approximate equivalent dose of these drugs is:

Mecamylamine	2.5 mg
Chlorisondamine	12.5 mg
Pentolinium	20.0 mg

Drug tolerance is common, requiring increments in dosage necessary in order to maintain postural hypotension. The duration of the action of drugs is increased when they are given together with a diuretic such as chlorothiazide. Thus, side effects can be decreased since the dosage of ganglionic blocking agents can be reduced.

RESERPINE

Reserpine, a prototype of several alkaloids present in *Rauwolfia serpentina* (Indian snakeroot), was introduced into Western medicine in the 1950's for its antihypertensive and tranquilizing properties. The drug causes almost complete depletion of catecholamines and serotonin in the central and peripheral nervous systems (Fig. 84). In animal experiments, it has been shown that the depletion of catecholamines in dose-dependent and maximal depletion occurs following the administration of 0.5 mg/kg (Bhagat, 1964). Larger doses exhibit no significantly greater effect.

The sensitivities of different organs to the depleting action of reserpine vary greatly (Carlsson *et al.*, 1957). Maximal depletion (90%) in the rat heart following a single dose of reserpine occurs at 4 hours (Bhagat, 1964).

TABLE XVI
Ganglionic Blockade vs Selective Sympathetic Inhibition

Predominant Tone Prior to Drug	Effect of Drug	
	Ganglionic Blocking Agents	Adrenergic Neuron Blocking Agents

Cardiovascular System

	Predominant Tone Prior to Drug	Ganglionic Blocking Agents	Adrenergic Neuron Blocking Agents
Arterioles	Sympathetic	Decrease in Arteriolar Tone Vasodilation; Decreased Peripheral Resistance; Increased Peripheral Flow; *Hypotension*; Blockade of Pressoreceptors (Reflex Adjustment)	Decrease in Arteriolar Tone Vasodilation; Decreased Peripheral Resistance; Increased Peripheral Flow; *Hypotension*; Blockade of Pressoreceptors (Reflex Adjustment)
Vein	Sympathetic	Decrease in Venous Tone; Increased Venous Capacity; Decreased Venous Return; Decreased Cardiac Output	Decrease in Venous Tone; Increased Venous Capacity; Decreased Venous Return; Decreased Cardiac Output
Heart	Parasympathetic	Increase in Heart Rate (Tachycardia)	Decrease in Heart Rate (Bradycardia)

Other Visceral Organs

	Predominant Tone Prior to Drug	Ganglionic Blocking Agents	Adrenergic Neuron Blocking Agents
G.I. tract	Parasympathetic	*Inhibition* of Parasympathetic Tone Resulting in Reduced G.I. Motility Reduced G.I. Secretion and Constipation	*Predominance* of Parasympathetic Tone Resulting in Increased G.I. Motility Increased Gastric Secretion and Diarrhea
		—	Nasal Congestion
iris	Parasympathetic	Mydriasis	Miosis
ciliary muscle	Parasympathetic	Cyclopegia	—
urinary bladder,	Parasympathetic	Retention of Urine in the Bladder	—
sexual organ	Parasympathetic	Impotence	Loss of Ejaculation without Loss of Potency

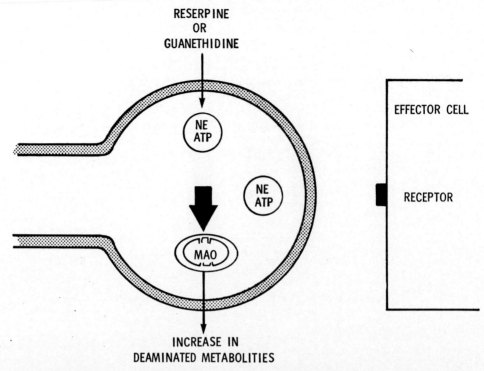

Figure 84. Schematic representation of the site of action of reserpine or guanethidine in the adrenergic neuron. Reserpine and guanethidine act on vesicles which are more deeply located in the neuron. The released norepinephrine is exposed to the action of monoamine oxidase. Thus norepinephrine leaves the nerve terminals as an inactivated deaminated metabolite.

In rat adrenals, the greatest depletion (50%) occurs only after three days (Cullingham and Mann, 1962).

The depletion of norepinephrine by reserpine is reduced by prior treatment of the animal with ganglionic blocking agents (Bhagat, 1963a), adrenergic neuron blocking agents (Bhagat, 1963a) and monoamine oxidase inhibitors (Bhagat, 1963b). The common factor in all of these experiments appears to be an inhibition of the spontaneous release by tonic impulses in the sympathetic nerves. Thus, it appears that tonic impulse traffic plays a role in the depleting action of reserpine (Hertting, *et al.,* 1962b; Weiner *et al.,* 1962; Bhagat, 1963a). The pharmacological consequences of this depletion are (a) impairment in the adrenergic nerve transmission, (b) the loss of action of those sympathomimetic amines, which are presumed to act indirectly by release of norepinephrine from the nerve ending, (c) hypotension, (d) sedation, (e) ptosis and (f) miosis.

Recent evidence indicates that minute quantities of reserpine are irreversibly bound in tissues with adrenergic innervation and that a linear relationship exists between the degree of norepinephrine depletion and the concentration of persistently bound reserpine. It has been demonstrated in rat heart that one molecule of persistently bound reserpine is associated with the depletion of about 500 norepinephrine molecules.

Effect on Retention of Norepinephrine

After administration of reserpine, the adrenergic neuron is not only depleted of its catecholamine, but the tissue also loses its capacity to take up norepinephrine. The onset of recovery of the capacity of the tissue to take up and retain small amounts of ^{3}H-norepinephrine occurs between 30 to 48 hours after reserpine (Bhagat and Shideman, 1964; Iversen *et al.*, 1965; Bhagat *et al.*, 1966). Also during this time, the nerve function recovers from the pharmacological effects of reserpine (Andén *et al.*, 1964; Andén and Henning, 1966). It seems that the time at which reserpine-induced inhibition of amine storage begins to disappear is very important, since at this time, most of the pharmacological effects of reserpine treatment have dissipated. The behavior of the animal is almost normal, in spite of the very low norepinephrine content of the tissue. The response to tyramine returns to normal (Bhagat *et al.*, 1966). All these findings imply that the normal function of the adrenergic system is possible in the presence of definite subnormal total catecholamine content in the tissue.

The coinciding effect of functional recovery, marks the onset of an increase in the endogenous norepinephrine level (Bhagat and Shideman, 1964). The recovery of these two factors, i.e. the uptake mechanism and endogenous norepinephrine levels, is due to formation and down transport of new granules from the cell bodies to the nerve terminals (Dahlström and Häggendal, 1966a,b). When down transport of new functioning amine storage granules was inhibited by ligation of the adrenergic nerve fiber in the reserpine pretreated rat, the recovery of the storage mechanism was markedly delayed.

Although reserpine interferes with the storage mechanism, it does not interfere with the transport of amines into the nerve terminals as does cocaine. As a consequence, the norepinephrine which enters the sympathetic neurons cannot be retained in the normal granule storage site and is rapidly metabolized by monoamine oxidase. This explains why there is no supersensitivity to norepinephrine after short-term treatment with reserpine. What little sensitization is observed is due to prolonged interruption of the normal impulse discharge of tonic impulses from the central nervous system to the effector organ. This supersensitivity is nonspecific, being equally pronounced in response to a variety of drugs.

It has been found that reserpine blocks the Mg^{++} and ATP-dependent uptake of dopamine and norepinephrine into the storage vesicles.

Effect of Reserpine on the Synthesis of Catecholamine

Reserpine can affect the rate of synthesis of norepinephrine by at least four mechanisms. First, it blocks the uptake of dopamine into the storage vesicles, the site of the β-hydroxylating enzyme. Thus the conversion of dopamine into norepinephrine is impaired. Next, it releases the norepinephrine from the storage vesicles into the cytoplasm, resulting in an increase in the free intraneuronal norepinephrine. This increase of intraneuronal norepinephrine would inhibit the tyrosine hydroxylase, and conversion of tyrosine to dopa would be reduced. Similarly, reserpine, by preventing the storage of norepinephrine in the storage granules, would increase the free intraneuronal norepinephrine. An increase of the end product, norepinephrine, would markedly inhibit the activity of tyrosine hydroxylase. Finally, with more prolonged treatment with reserpine, the tyrosine hydroxylase activity is increased, and thereby the rate of synthesis of norepinephrine is increased. The enhanced tyrosine hydroxylase activity is due to a prolonged reflex increase in the sympathoadrenal activity as a consequence of reserpine-induced impairment of postganglionic sympathetic transmission.

Effect on Cardiovascular System

When reserpine is injected (2.5 mg, intramuscularly) in a normal person, the blood pressure falls within two hours. This is due to the depletion of catecholamine from its stores in the postganglionic nerve endings. The norepinephrine released from the storage granules into the axoplasm is exposed to the action of monoamine oxidase in the mitochondria which are present in the nerves. This norepinephrine leaves the nerve terminals as an inactive deaminated metabolite. Thus, there is an increase in catecholamine metabolites in the urine. In animal experiments intravenous administration of reserpine may cause transient elevation of blood pressure.

In a patient with severe hypertension, administration of reserpine causes a fall in blood pressure. This antihypertensive action is not due to tranquillizing properties since it has been observed that reserpine, in combination with thiazide diuretics, is more effective in lowering blood pressure than would be expected from its sedative effects alone.

Although it interferes with peripheral neurotransmission, it does not produce postural hypotension. In this respect it has advantages over ganglionic blocking and adrenergic neuron blocking agents.

When reserpine is given orally, there is a delay of several days before a significant effect is achieved.

This hypotensive condition is due to a decrease in peripheral resistance. Cardiac output remains unchanged or is slightly increased.

Side Effects

Due to decreased sympathetic activity
A) peripheral nervous system
   bradycardia
   aggravation of peptic ulcers

increased gastrointestinal motility

miosis

nasal stuffiness

All these are due to parasympathetic predominance as a result of depletion of catecholamines.

B) Central nervous system

drowsiness

lethargy

depression

Due to depression several patients have attempted suicide. Reserpine
enhances central nervous system depressant action of barbiturates and
alcohol. Syrosingopine produces fewer depressant actions in relation to its
antihypertensive action.

Preparation and the Mode of Administration

Reserpine is available in tablets containing 0.1, 0.25, 0.5, and 1 mg and
ampules containing 2.5 mg/ml in sizes of 2 and 10 ml. Syrosingopine is
available in tablets containing 1 mg. Rauwolfia (root) is available in
tablets of 50 and 100 mg.

Reserpine is taken in doses of 0.25 mg two or three times a day by mouth.
Syrosingopine is used in doses of 0.5 to 1 mg orally. It is not advisable to
administer these drugs parenterally.

Reserpine 0.1 mg a day in combination with thiazide is sufficient and is
less apt to cause side effects.

General Comments

1. The patient should be warned that he might get drowsy while driving.
2. Reserpine use should be avoided in the patient who shows any
   tendency toward depression.
3. Some patients may get nasal stuffiness during reserpine therapy. It
   is wise to stop treatment until it clears.
4. Patients should be warned about disturbing after-midnight dreams.
   The dreams are not nightmares but may sometimes be unpleasant.
   The use of the drug should be discontinued temporarily or its dose
   should be reduced.
5. Reserpine enhances gastric secretion, which may cause actual ulcers,
   and sometimes there is an increase in bowel motility. Its use should
   be avoided in patients with a history of ulcer problems.

ALPHA METHYLDOPA

α-Methyldopa (Aldomet) was introduced as an antihypertensive drug
on the basis of the observation that it competitively inhibits dopa decarboxylase *in vitro,* thereby inhibiting the conversion of dopa to dopamine.
It was assumed that this inhibition of synthesis of norepinephrine would

cause transmission failure in adrenergic nerves, decrease in sympathetic tone and fall in blood pressure. In the human body, dopa decarboxylase is present in such great quantities that it would be difficult to inhibit its activities with therapeutic doses. Furthermore, dopa decarboxylase is not a rate limiting enzyme and it cannot inhibit the rate of synthesis of catecholamines effectively. It was found, however, that the drug is taken up in the adrenergic neuron, and decarboxylated in the cytoplasm to α-methyl dopamine. Storage vesicles take up α-methyl-dopamine where it is β-hydroxylated to α-methyl norepinephrine. The presence of the α-methyl group makes the amine immune to the action of monoamine oxidase, hence it accumulates in the adrenergic neuron. α-methyl norepinephrine displaces the norepinephrine from its storage site and acts as a false neurotransmitter. Since its potency is lower than that of norepinephrine, decreased sympathetic activity results. Recent observations, however, have shown that α-methyl norepinephrine is as potent and effective as norepinephrine. It appears that this false transmitter might reduce blood pressure by being more slowly released from the nerves than norepinephrine.

Mechanism of action of adrenergic blockade by α-methyl dopa as compared with reserpine or guanethidine is presented in Table XVII.

Although α-methyldopa cannot inhibit dopa decarboxylase *in vivo* it may alter the rate of synthesis of norepinephrine in several ways. Its metabolites, α-methyl dopamine and α-methyl norepinephrine, may compete with the tetrahydropteridine cofactor for the reduced enzyme tyrosine hydroxylase and inhibit the conversion of tyrosine to dopa resulting in a diminished synthesis. α-Methyl dopamine may compete with dopamine for the site of synthesis of norepinephrine so that less dopamine may be converted to norepinephrine. Finally, the α-methyl norepinephrine formed may displace the norepinephrine from its storage site into the cytoplasm, resulting in increased free intraneuronal norepinephrine and, consequently, increase in the end-product inhibition of tyrosine hydroxylase.

When α-methyldopa is given to patients with essential hypertension, cardiac output falls slightly at a time when peripheral vascular resistance reduces significantly. Thus, α-methyldopa lowers blood pressure primarily by reducing peripheral vascular resistance. In this respect, it differs from guanethidine. The antihypertensive response to guanethidine is characterized by a significant reduction in cardiac output, while peripheral vascular resistance remains practically unchanged. The antihypertensive effect of α-methyldopa is greater when the patient is in an erect position than when the patient assumes a supine position. During the antihypertensive effect of α-methyldopa, renal blood flow is maintained or enhanced. Consequently, there is minimal depression of the glomerular filtration rate. Accordingly, α-methyldopa has been of particular value in the treatment of patients who require immediate reduction of the blood pressure but at the same time have renal functional impairment, and in patients with renal hypertension. The patient can be maintained on α-methyldopa for

TABLE XVII

MECHANISM OF ACTION OF ADRENERGIC BLOCKADE BY ANTIHYPERTENSIVE DRUGS

Drug	Acts Through a Metabolite?	Depletes Endogenous NE?	Blocks Neuronal Function Before Depletion?	Does the Active Compound Accumulate in Nerve Endings	Is Drug Released by Nerve Impulses?	Causes Supersensitivity to NE?
α-methyl-dopa	yes (α-mne)*	yes	no	yes α-mne	yes α-mne	no
Guanethidine	no	yes	yes	yes	yes	yes
Reserpine	no	yes	no	no	no	no

*α-mne = α-methyl norepinephrine

TABLE XVIII

COMPARISON OF THE EFFECTS OF ANTIHYPERTENSIVE DRUGS

	α-Methyl dopa	Guanethidine	Reserpine
Heart rate	Decreased	Decreased	Slightly decreased
Cardiac output	Unchanged	Decreased	Unchanged
Total peripheral resistance	Decreased	Little or no decrease	Decreased
Blood pressure	Fall	Fall	Fall
Renal blood flow	No significant change	Decreased	No significant change
Glomerular filtration rate	No significant change	Decreased	No significant change
Renal vascular resistance	Decreased	No significant change	Decrease
Degree of postural hypotension	Moderate	Marked	Not Significant
Central effects	Mild Sedation	No significant effect	Serious depression

1 to 2 weeks. This period is enough to permit readjustment of renal hemodynamics. Thereafter, the patient can be put on other potent antihypertensive therapy. The comparison of the α-methyl dopa with guanthidine and reserpine is presented in Table XVIII.

Preparations

Methyldopa is available in tablets containing 250 mg of the drug. Methyldopate (α-methyl ester hydrochloride) is available for intravenous injection. The 5 ml ampule contains 250 mg of the drug.

The drug is absorbed well when taken orally and begins to reduce blood pressure within the first 24 hours of intake. The beginning dose is 250 mg two to three times a day. The dose can be increased to 500 mg four times a day.

Side Effects

Sedation, depression
Dry mouth
Enlargement of breast
Lactation
Nightmares
Febrile reaction
Alterations in hepatic function
Tiredness
Some patients receiving α-methyldopa develop positive direct Coombs tests.

General Comments

1. α-methyldopa is considered intermediate between mild and strong hypotensive agents. Its importance lies in its greater ability to lower blood pressure in the supine position than the other antihypertensive drugs.
2. α-methyldopa is used in patients for whom reserpine is contraindicated because they give a history of depression.
3. α-methyldopa should be used in combination with thiazide diuretics. Its effects are potentiated by this combination.
4. Postural hypotension is considerably less than with guanethidine or ganglionic blocking agents.
5. α-methyldopa is used in patients with renal failure or in hypertension with renal origin. In patients with renal failure, this drug is very beneficial because it is not excreted by the kidney, and therefore it accumulates and causes severe hypotension.
6. Tolerance rarely occurs.

GUANETHIDINE

Guanethidine is a very potent antihypertensive agent, and it has very complex effects on the adrenergic neuron:

TYRAMINE-LIKE EFFECT—When administered intravenously it causes a transient rise in the blood pressure. This is due to release of catecholamine from tissue stores. When norepinephrine stores are depleted by pretreatment with reserpine, there is no rise in blood pressure after guanethidine. The response is restored following infusion of norepinephrine. This phenomenon has been interpreted as a *refilling* of the depleted stores and a subsequent release by guanethidine.

ADRENERGIC NEURON BLOCKING EFFECT. Following a transient rise in blood pressure, guanethidine administration causes adrenergic nerve blockade. Thus, guanethidine prevents the release of norepinephrine from the postganglionic nerve endings. This is not due to any interference with the conduction of nerve impulses nor to the depletion of catecholamines. This early neuronal blockade occurs at a time when catecholamines are not yet depleted in the nerve. Since injected norepinephrine is able to exert its effects, adrenergic receptors are still functional.

RESERPINE-LIKE EFFECT. Finally, guanethidine causes depletion of catecholamine stores, thereby leading to a blockade of neurotransmission. The effect is similar to that of reserpine (Fig. 84). As would be expected, indirectly acting amines lose their effectiveness after guanethidine.

COCAINE-LIKE EFFECT. Not only catecholamines are depleted after guanethidine, but also there is impairment in the uptake mechanism. Therefore, as after cocaine, response to injected catecholamine is potentiated, because norepinephrine may reach higher concentrations at the receptors of the effector organs (Fig. 85).

Effect on Cardiovascular System

Administration of guanethidine causes a fall in blood pressure. This fall in blood pressure is mostly due to a significant reduction in cardiac output. The peripheral vascular resistance remains essentially unchanged. Due to reduced cardiac output, renal plasma flow and glomerular filtration rate are reduced. It causes bradycardia, probably through blockade of sympathetic impulses to the sino-atrial node.

In contrast to reserpine it causes severe orthostatic hypotension. The reason for this difference between the two is difficult to explain. Some people believe guanethidine may have a greater effect on capacitance vessels while reserpine has effects on resistance vessels.

The antihypertensive effect of guanethidine can be reversed by certain tricyclic antidepressants such as desimipramine and amphetamine. Amphetamine probably competes with guanethidine for uptake into the adrenergic neuron. On the other hand, desimipramine blocks the uptake of guanethidine into the adrenergic neuron.

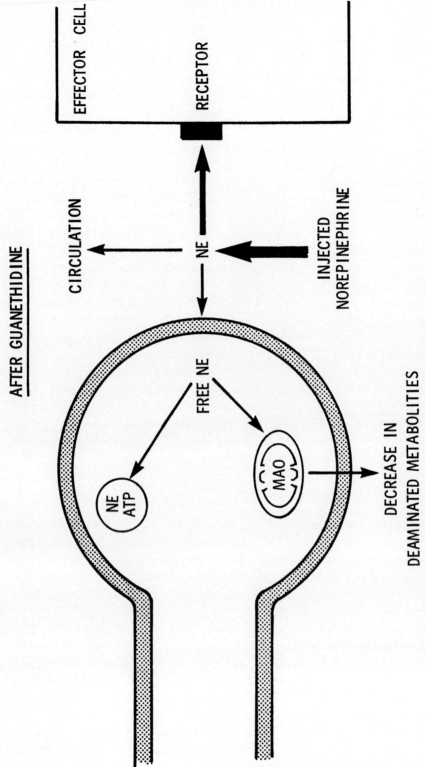

Figure 85. Normally most of the injected norepinephrine is taken up into nerve terminals, some diffuses away and very little acts on the receptors of the effector organ. After administration of guanethidine transport of norepinephrine into the nerve terminal is impaired so that more of the injected norepinephrine is available on the adrenergic receptors.

Preparation

Guanethidine is available in tablets containing 10 and 20 mg of the drug. Since the drug can aggravate hypertensive emergencies, it is not administered parenterally. When taken orally, it is fairly well absorbed from the gastro-intestinal tract and is excreted largely in an unchanged form. Usual starting dose is 10 mg/day. The onset of action is 5 to 7 days. In the case of severe hypertension, the dose can be increased to 25 mg per day.

Side Effects

A number of the adverse effects of guanethidine are due to an unopposed activity of the parasympathetic nervous system and to the reduced activity of the sympathetic nervous system. The main side effects are:

1. diarrhea
2. aggravation of peptic ulcer
3. parotid pain
4. nasal stuffiness
5. failure of ejaculation
6. nocturia
7. lowering intraoccular pressure
8. general weakness
9. water retention

General Comments

1) Guanethidine is considered the most potent of all the antihypertensive agents. Its use is suggested in patients who maintain a diastolic pressure of 120 mm Hg or greater because of its side effects.

2) Diarrhea is a frequent side effect. It manifests itself as frequency of bowel habit rather than loose stool. Bowel frequency is dose related and can be cured with atropine like drugs (0.4 mg per day or more as needed). Some patients complain of explosive and uncontrollable bowel evacuation, usually as a gastrocolic reflex after eating when they would normally have a bowel movement.

3) It has a strange effect on male sexual function, preventing ejaculation without affecting erection. The failure of ejaculation can be reversed only by reduction in guanethidine dosage or else discontinuation of the drug.

4) Unlike the ganglionic blocking agents, guanethidine does not cause parasympathetic blockade, and therefore it does not produce side effects such as constipation, dryness of mouth and blurring of vision, so common with the use of ganglionic blocking agents.

5) Guanethidine causes a marked hypotension when the patient is in the erect position.

6) The patient should be warned against syncopal episode; he should exert caution when getting out of bed.

7) Since renal plasma flow and glomerular filtration rate are reduced after guanethidine, it should be used with caution in hypertensive patients with renal insufficiency; dosage must be regulated with care.

8) Guanethidine does not cross the blood brain barrier and therefore does not cause sedation and depression. Its use is desirable in patients with a history of depression.

9) It is preferable that it should be used in combination with a diuretic or α-methyldopa.

10) When higher doses are used, it may be given in divided doses.

11) Tolerance does develop to guanethidine.

12) Interaction of drugs such as antihistamines, monoamine oxidase inhibitors, and methylphenidate (Ritalin®) with guanethidine emphasize the need for caution in the use of other agents concomitantly. Co-administration of guanethidine and monoamine oxidase inhibitor may result in dangerous paradoxical pressor reactions.

MONOAMINE OXIDASE INHIBITORS

Norepinephrine released intraneuronally into the cytoplasm is deaminated by monoamine oxidase present in the mitochondria. When monoamine oxidase is inhibited, levels of norepinephrine in various organs are elevated. One of the surprising effects of monoamine oxidase inhibitors is that they cause a fall in blood pressure. The mechanism of this antihypertensive action is not yet clearly understood. One of the most attractive explanations for the antihypertensive action of inhibitors of monoamine oxidase is that inhibition of the enzyme allows the accumulation of octopamine in the sympathetic nerve endings, and is subsequently released as a false neurotransmitter.

Ordinarily, tyramine is formed in the body by the decarboxylation of tyrosine. Since tyramine is a good substrate for monoamine oxidase, it is destroyed. After inhibition of monoamine oxidase, it is not destroyed; instead, it enters the sympathetic neuron in the storage vesicle where it is β-hydroxylated to octopamine.

Since octopamine potency is less than that of norepinephrine, there is a decrease in sympathetic function. This fact may account for the low blood pressure achieved in hypertensive patients treated with MAO inhibitors.

Pargyline hydrochloride (Eutonyl®) is the most useful MAO inhibitor. Its antihypertensive potency is equivalent to guanethidine and the ganglion-blocking agents.

It decreases peripheral vascular resistance. Renal vascular resistance is only slightly reduced; therefore, renal blood flow and glomerular filtration rate are not significantly affected. Cardiac output is not significantly changed.

Side Effects

orthostatic hypotension
gastrointestinal disturbance

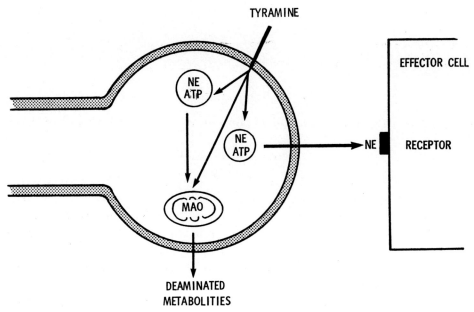

Figure 86. *Schematic representation of the site of action of tyramine in the adrenergic neuron.* Tyramine displaces the norepinephrine from its storage site. The release of norepinephrine from vesicles occurs throughout the cytoplasm of the nerve terminals, both deep and close to the synaptic cleft. Some norepinephrine leaves the nerve terminal; however, substantial amounts of norepinephrine are oxidatively deaminated within the neuron. Tyramine itself is a good substrate for monoamine oxidase and part of the injected amine is destroyed by the monoamine oxidase.

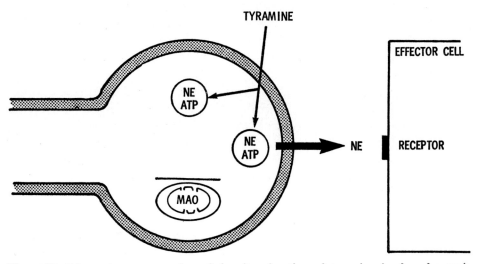

Figure 87. Schematic representation of the site of action of tyramine in the adrenergic neuron after inhibition of monoamine oxidase. Tyramine is a good substrate of monoamine oxidase. As soon as tyramine is taken up by the nerve ending, a considerable amount of it is removed by monoamine oxidase. When monoamine oxidase is inhibited by prior treatment of animals with pargyline, the amount of norepinephrine released by tyramine is increased.

insomnia
dry mouth
weight gain
impotence or inability to ejaculate

Preparation

Pargyline is available in tablets containing 10, 25 and 50 mg of drug.

General Comments

1) The recommended dose is 10 to 25 mg daily. It takes 2 to 3 weeks before maximum effect is achieved. After 2 to 3 weeks, the dose may be increased to 50 mg. The maximum dose is 50 mg three times a day. The effect is cumulative and remains long after the therapy is discontinued. In some patients tolerance has been noted.
2) Its efficacy is improved when given in combination with thiazide diuretic drugs.
3) It can be used in patients who for one reason or another cannot tolerate other drugs, e.g. guanethidine, methyldopa, reserpine, or do not respond adequately to these drugs.
4) Since pargyline is an antidepressant it may alleviate psychic depression. Therefore it is useful in patients with a history of depression.
5) Its use in the hypertensive patient with obesity may create a problem in weight control.
6) It is contraindicated in patients with severe renal failure or in those suspected of pheochromocytoma.
7) The drug interacts with many foods and other drugs. Certain types of cheeses, wines and beer containing high levels of pressor amine tyramine pose a problem in that hypertensive crisis may be precipitated. The mechanism of this untoward response relates to the release of norepinephrine from the post-ganglionic sympathetic nerve endings by tyramine (Fig. 86). Ordinarily, when food or beer is taken, tyramine present in the food is destroyed in the body by monoamine oxidase. After inhibition of monoamine oxidase by pargyline, tyramine is not destroyed and may cause an enhanced release of norepinephrine resulting in a greater rise in blood pressure (Fig. 87).

DIURETIC

The thiazide diuretics are considered valuable therapeutic agents in the control of hypertension. It has been estimated that one-half of all hypertensive patients with a diastolic pressure of 115 mm Hg or less can be relieved by diuretic drugs alone.

The natriuretic and diuretic effects of the thiazide drugs are mainly due to their ability to inhibit the reabsorption of sodium in the renal tubules, probably at a distal site. In addition, most of the thiazide diuretics are

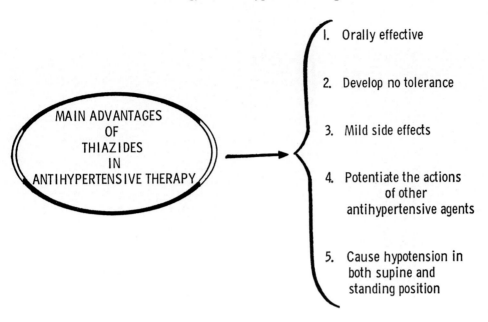

MAIN ADVANTAGES
OF
THIAZIDES
IN
ANTIHYPERTENSIVE THERAPY

1. Orally effective

2. Develop no tolerance

3. Mild side effects

4. Potentiate the actions
   of other
   antihypertensive agents

5. Cause hypotension in
   both supine and
   standing position

weak inhibitors of the enzyme carbonic anhydrase, resulting in an additional effect, to enhance sodium excretion.

The antihypertensive effect of these agents is in proportion to their natriuretic effect; the mode of action to lower the blood pressure of the hypertensive patient, however, is not yet known. In normotensive patients, these drugs do not effect the blood pressure. The antihypertensive effects of oral diuretic treatment are associated with sodium loss and apparently not to any direct vasodilator effect. This may not be the whole explanation: it may, indeed, prove to have no part at all in the true explanation. Diazoxide is a drug with very much the same antihypertensive action as chlorothiazide; in some cases, it is more useful than the latter drug because it may restore the hypotensive response to drugs to which the patient has become adapted. Yet, diazoxide causes retention of sodium and water to such an extent that oedema sometimes develops.

At the initial stages of thiazide treatment, the blood pressure reduction is associated with a decrease in plasma and extracellular fluid volumes resulting in a decrease in cardiac output. The hypotensive action of the thiazide agents at this point is attributed to the reduced cardiac output, since peripheral vascular resistance has been shown to be elevated. This is unlikely on explanation for the hypotensive effect of these drugs when administered for a prolonged period. Following long-term administration of these drugs, the plasma volume and extracellular fluid volume return to normal values, though there is no concomitant return of the blood pressure. Moreover, if the plasma volume of a patient who is being successfully treated with chlorothiazide is increased by an infusion of dextran, there is no marked increase in blood pressure. The hypotensive response persists as the result of a secondary reduction in peripheral vascular resistance. The

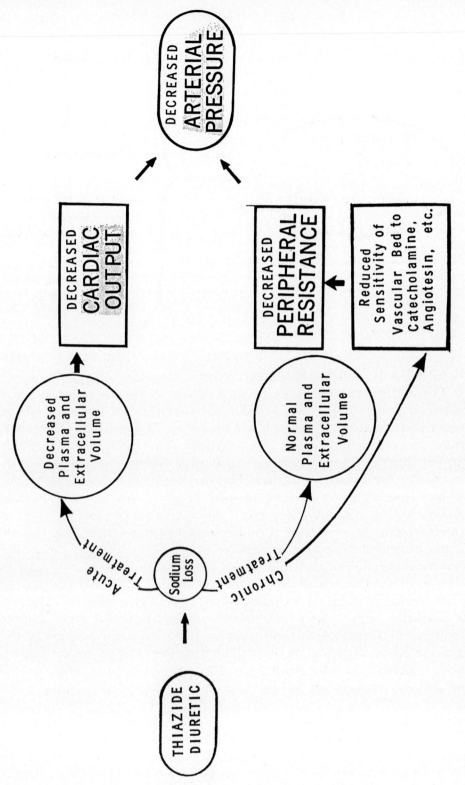

Figure 88. *Schematic Representation of the Mechanism of Antihypertensive Action of Thiazide Diuretics*

explanation for the decrease in vascular resistance is not known. It has been suggested that a reduced sodium content in smooth muscle cells following thiazide therapy reduces their sensitivity to catecholamines and angiotensin.

Thus, it appears that shifts in the distribution of water and electrolytes, especially sodium and possibly also potassium, may be an integral part of the hypertensive process.

The hypotensive action of the thiazide agents is more specific than most other antihypertensive drugs, since they lower blood pressure primarily in patients with hypertension rather than in all individuals, and then, only to levels that are above normal. Although the oral thiazide diuretics may be effective when administered alone, their greatest usefulness in the treatment of hypertensive disease is in enhancing the hypotensive effectiveness of other blood pressure-lowering drugs. This combination permits excellent control of blood pressure in many instances where this was not possible previously. Moreover, the antihypertensive effect can be accomplished with relatively low doses of the various antihypertensive agents, and hence, with minimum toxicity and few side effects. Thus, rauwolfia causes only a mild reduction in blood pressure when used alone; but, when used in combination with a thiazide derivative, it lowers blood pressure to a more significant degree. The combination of guanethidine and a thiazide diuretic agent has been reported to decrease the blood pressure effectively in more than 90 percent of hypertensive patients. The synergistic, hypotensive effect of the thiazide agents in combination with all other antihypertensive agents has made them the most popular and most prescribed of the antihypertensive drugs. They may be used alone, but for greatest effect are combined with a second antihypertensive agent, mostly with a sympathetic blocking agent. There is little advantage of one thiazide preparation over another except perhaps in terms of cost or greater convenience in dosage schedules, which the longer-acting preparations may provide. The drug is prescribed for the morning hours so that the diuretic effects will be most prominent while the patient is awake.

The mechanism of the action of diuretics is summarized in Figure 88.

Side Effects

The thiazide agents usually are well tolerated. Occasional complaints include nausea, gastric irritation, headache, fatigue, muscle cramps, and weakness, probably due to electrolyte abnormalities. In some patients, skin rashes, leukopenia, thrombocytopenia purpura, and petechiae have been reported, and the use of drugs should be discontinued temporarily. Other rare side effects include pancreatitis, photosensitivity, and intrahepatic cholestatic jaundice.

HYDRALAZINE

In 1950, it was found that the hydralazine-like drugs had the unusual ability of both lowering blood pressure and increasing renal blood flow.

Following administration, blood pressure falls in both normotensive and hypertensive patients. There is always a delay of about 10 minutes before the blood pressure falls, even after intravenous administration.

Effect on Cardiovascular System

Hydralazine has a stimulant effect on the heart, resulting in tachycardia and increased cardiac output. It is a nonspecific inhibitor of a variety of vasoconstrictor stimuli such as histamine, barium chloride, vasopressin, pressor amines, and sympathetic tone. It acts directly on arteriolar smooth muscle to decrease peripheral resistance resulting in vasodilatation. Pharmacodynamic studies in man confirm that blood pressure is lowered by a decrease in peripheral vascular resistance due to arteriolar vasodilation.

Thus, hydralazine causes an increase in cardiac output which is associated with an increased cardiac rate and stroke volume at the time when the peripheral resistance is reduced and the blood pressure lowered. It, therefore, seems to exert a favorable effect, more on the diastolic than the systolic pressure. There is evidence that renal arterioles are especially affected; thus, renal blood flow is preserved unless the blood pressure fall is marked (Fig. 89).

Preparations and Mode of Administration

Hydralazine is available in tablets containing 10, 25, 50, and 100 mg of the drug. Ampules of hydralazine contain 20 mg of the drug/1 ml.

Hydralazine may be given by mouth or by intramuscular injection. The starting oral dose may be 10 mg three or four times daily. The dose may be increased at weekly intervals, but should not exceed 100 mg four times daily. Tolerance may develop to the hypotensive action of the drug, but it disappears when drug is discontinued for a week or so. The injectable form, intramuscular or intravenous, is best reserved for hypertensive emergencies.

Toxic Effect

The side effects of hydralazine consist of headache, palpitations, nausea and vomiting, diarrhea, nasal congestion, conjunctivitis, drug fever, skin rash, peripheral neuropathy, and bone marrow suppression.

The cardiac stimulatory effect of hydralazine may provoke anginal pain and myocardial infarction in patients with prior coronary artery disease.

The most notorious effect of prolonged hydralazine therapy is the development of a polyarthritis that resembles rheumatoid arthritis and may progress to a stage of lupus erythematosis. In a few instances symptoms did not entirely disappear, even when the drug was discontinued in the treatment of hypertensive crises. At any rate, this potential hazard greatly reduces the effectiveness of hydralazine. The lupus-like syndrome has never

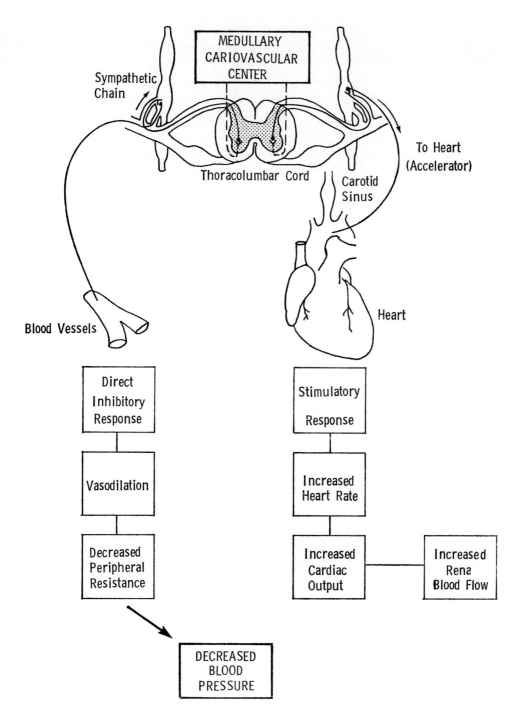

Figure 89. *Schematic Representation of the Mechanism of Antihypertensive Action of Hydralazine*

been produced following short-term intravenous or intramuscular administration.

General Comments

1. Hydralazine is a potent antihypertensive agent, and it has been recommended for the management of essential hypertension and early forms of the malignant disease. It finds application also in acute hypertensive episodes.

2. Since it increases renal blood flow in an association with an increase in cardiac output, it is very useful in the treatment of patients with renal dysfunction.

3. When hydralazine is being used in conjunction with thiazide and reserpine, very few side effects develop.

4. The complications of angina and tachycardia are more serious and much more common. When used in combination with either rauwolfia or guanethidine, both of which have bradycardiac effects, the tachycardia produced by hydralazine may be neutralized and therefore the risk to the patient with angina diminished.

5. There may be some headache and occasionally the headache is severe. It was claimed at one time that headache was an initial symptom in some 40 percent of patients given hydralazine but it disappears spontaneously as the treatment is continued. In some patients headache can be continuous and incapacitating as long as the drug is taken, and the drug may have to be discontinued.

6. It seems advisable to warn the patient that weakness, palpitation, nausea, and, less commonly, numbness in the extremities, flushing, and conjunctival inflammation may occur.

7. Hydralazine is a drug of choice for treatment of hypertension in patients whose plasma catecholamines and plasma renin activity are within the normal range. It can restore blood pressure to normal levels without depressing sympathetic activity below normal. Concomitant administration of propanolol (80 to 200 mg daily, orally) with hydralazine will prevent sympathetic reflex response of hypertensive patient to blood pressure reduction that increases cardiac output inappropriately.

REFERENCES

Abraham, A.: *Microscopic Innervation of the Heart and Blood Vessels in Vertebrates* aline in sympathetic nerves. *Prog Brain Res, 31*:21-32, 1969.

Abrams, W.B.: The Mechanisms of action of antihypertensive drugs. *Dis Chest, 55:* 149-159, 1969.

Ahlquist, R.P.: A study of the adrenotropic receptors. *Am J Physiol, 153:* 586-600, 1948.

Alexander, R.S.: Tonic and reflex functions of medullary sympathetic cardiovascular centers. *J Neurophysiol, 9:* 205-217, 1946.

Andén, N. and Henning, M.: Adrenergic nerve function, noradrenaline level and noradrenaline uptake in cat nictitating membrane after reserpine treatment. *Acta Physiol Scand, 67:* 498-504, 1966.

Andén, N., Magnusson, T. and Waldeck, B.: Correlation between noradrenaline uptake and adrenergic nerve function after reserpine treatment. *Life Sci, 3:* 19-25, 1964.

Andén, N.E., Carlsson, A. and Häggendal, J.: Adrenergic mechanism. *Ann Rev Pharmac, 9:* 119-134, 1969.

Angelkos, E.T., Fuxe, K. and Torchiana, M.: Chemical and histochemical evaluation of the distribution of catecholamines in the rabbit and guinea pig hearts. *Acta Physiol Scand, 59:* 184-192, 1963.

Avakain, O.V. and Gillespie, J.S.: Uptake of noradrenaline by adrenergic nerves. Smooth muscle and connective tissue in isolated perfused arteries and its correlation with vasoconstrictor response. *Br J Pharmacol, 32:* 168-184, 1968.

Axelrod, J.: Dopamine-β-Hydroxylase: Regulation of its synthesis and release from nerve terminal. *Pharmac Rev, 24:* 233-243, 1972.

Axelrod, J. and Kopin, I.J.: The uptake, storage, release and metabolism of noradrenaline in sympathetic nerves. *Prog Brain Res, 31:* 1969.

Axelrod, J. and Tomchick, R.: Enzymatic o-methylation of epinephrine and other catechols. *J Biol Chem, 233:* 702-705, 1958.

Axelrod, J. and Weinshilboum, R.: Catecholamines. *New Eng J Med, 285:* (5), 237-242, 1972.

Axelrod, J., Hertting, G. and Patrick, R.W.: Inhibition of H[3]-norepinephrine by monoamine oxidase inhibitors. *J Pharmacol Exp Ther, 134:* 325-328, 1961.

Axelrod, J., Hertting, G. and Potter, L.T.: Effect of drugs on the uptake and release of H[3]-norepinephrine in the rat heart. *Nature* (London), *194:* 297, 1962.

Barnett, A. and Benforado, J.N.: The nicotine effect of choline esters and of nicotine in guinea pig atria. *J Pharmacol Exp Ther, 152:* 29-36, 1966.

Bayliss, W.M.: On the local reaction of the arterial walls to changes of internal pressure. *J Physiol* (London), *28:* 220-231, 1902.

Beaven, J.A. and Verity, M.A.: Sympathetic nerve-free vascular muscle. *J. Pharmacol Exp Ther, 157:* 117-124, 1967.

Beaven, J.A., Osher, J.V. and Beaven, R.D.: Distribution of bound norepinephrine in the arterial wall. *Eur J Pharmacol, 5:* 299-301, 1969.

Bergstrom, S., Carlson, L.A., and Weeks, J.R.: The prostaglandins: A family of biologically active lipids. *Pharmac Rev, 20:* 1-48, 1968.

185

Berneis, K.H., DePrada, M. and Pletscher, A.: Micelle formation between 5-hydroxytryptamine and adenosine triphosphate in platelet storage organelles. *Science, 165:* 913-914, 1969a.

Berneis, K.H., Pletscher, A. and DaPrada, P.: Metal-dependent aggregation of biogenic amines: A hypothesis for their storage and release. *Nature* (London), *224:* 281-282, 1969b.

Berneis, K.H., Pletscher, A. and DaPrada, M.: Phase separation in solutions of noradrenaline and adenosine triphosphate: influence of bivalent cations and drugs. *Br J Pharmacol, 39:* 382-389, 1970.

Berti, F. and Shore, P.A.: A kinetic analysis of drugs that inhibit the adrenergic neuronal membrane amine pump. *Biochem Pharmacol, 16:* 2091-2094, 1967.

Bertler, A. and Rosengren, E.: Occurrence and distribution of catecholamines in brain. *Acta Physiol Scand, 47:* 350-361, 1959.

Bhagat, B.: The effect of adrenergic neuron blocking agents on the release and uptake of catecholamines by the rat heart. *Arch Int Pharmacodyn, 146:* 231-237, 1963a.

Bhagat, B.: The effect of various monoamine oxidase inhibitors on the catecholamine content of rat heart. *Arch Int Pharmacodyn, 146:* 65-72, 1963b.

Bhagat, B.: Effect of reserpine on cardiac catecholamines. *Life Sci, 3:* 1361-1370, 1964.

Bhagat, B.: The influence of sympathetic nervous activity on cardiac catecholamine levels. *J Pharmacol Exp Ther, 157:* 74-80, 1967.

Bhagat, B.: Effect of chronic cold stress on catecholamine levels in rat brain. *Psychopharmacologia* (Berlin), *16:* 1-4, 1969a.

Bhagat, B.: Increased turnover rate of norepinephrine (NE) in rat brain induced by repeated administration of nicotine. *Pharmacologist, 11* (2): 250, 1969b.

Bhagat, B.: Role of adrenal hormones in the synthesis of noradrenaline in cardiac sympathetic neurones. *Br J Pharmacol, 37:* 34-40, 1969c.

Bhagat, B.: Effect of chronic administration of nicotine on storage and synthesis of noradrenaline in rat brain. *Br J Pharmacol, 38:* 86-92, 1970.

Bhagat, B. and Shideman, F.E.: Reflection of cardiac catecholamines in the rat: importance of the adrenal medulla and synthesis from precursors. *J Pharmacol Exp Ther, 143:* 77-81, 1964.

Bhagat, B. and Ragland, R.: Effect of infusion of metaraminol on the response of reserpine-pretreated spinal cats to tyramine and to noradrenaline. *Br J Pharmacol, 27:* 506-513, 1966.

Bhagat, B., Bhattacharya, I.C. and Dhalla, N.S.: Retention of exogenous norepinephrine and recovery of the responses to tyramine and 1, 1-dimethyl-4-phenylpiperazinium iodide after reserpine. *J Pharmacol Exp Ther, 153:* 434-439, 1966.

Bhagat, B., Bovell, G. and Robinson, I.M.: Influence of cocaine on the uptake of ^{3}H-norepinephrine and on the responses of isolated guinea pig atria to sympathomimetic amines. *J Pharmacol Exp Ther, 155:* 472-478, 1967.

Bhagat, B., Burke, W.J. and Davis, J.W.: Effect of reserpine on the activity of adrenal enzymes involved in the synthesis of adrenaline. *Br J Pharmacol, 43:* 819-827, 1971.

Bhagat, B., Dhalla, N.S., Ginn, D., LaMontagne, A.E. and Montier, A.D.: Modification by prostaglandin E_2 (PGE_2) of the response of guinea pig isolated vas deferentia and atria to adrenergic stimuli. *Br J Pharmacol, 44:* 689-698, 1972.

Biglieri, E.A.: Hypertension with primary and secondary hyperaldosteronism. *Postgrad Med, 52:* (3), 78-82, 1972.

Bjorklund, A., Cegrell, L., Falck, B., Ritzen, M. and Rosengren, E.: Dopamine containing cells in sympathetic ganglia. *Acta Physiol Scand, 78:* 334-339, 1970.

Blaschko, H.: The specific action of L-dopa decarboxylase. *J Physiol* (London), *96:* 5-51, 1939.

Bogdanski, D.F. and Brodie, B.B.: Role of sodium and potassium ions in storage of norepinephrine by sympathetic nerve endings. *Life Sci, 5:* 1563-1569, 1966.

Bogdanski, D.F. and Brodie, B.B.: The effect of inorganic ions on the storage and uptake of H³-norepinephrine by rat heart slices. *J Pharmacol Exp Ther, 165:* 181-189, 1969.

Bohr, D.F.: Adrenergic receptors in coronary arteries. *Ann NY Acad Sci, 139:* 799-807, 1967.

Brodie, B.B., Costa, E.E., D Labac, A., Neff, N.H. and Smookler, H.H.: Application of steady state kinetics to the estimation of synthesis rate and turnover time of tissue catecholamines. *J Pharmacol Exp Ther., 154:* 493-499, 1966.

Brunjes, S., Johns, V.J., Jr. and Crane, M.G.: Pheochromocytoma: postoperative shock and blood volume. *New Eng J Med, 262:*393-396, 1960.

Burnstock, G. and Holman, M.E.: Spontaneous potentials at sympathetic nerve endings in smooth muscle. *J Physiol* (London), *160:* 446-460, 1962.

Carlsson, A.: Pharmacology of the Sympathetic Nervous System. In: *Antihypertensive Therapy,* F. Gross (Ed.), New York, Springer-Verlag, pp. 5-14, 1966.

Carlsson, A. and Lindquist, M.: *In vivo* decarboxylation of α-methyl metatyrosine. *Acta Physiol Scand, 54:* 37-99, 1962.

Carlsson, A., Rosengren, E., Bertler, A. and Nilsson, J.: Effect of Reserpine on the Metabolism of Catecholamines. In Garattini, S., and Ghettis, V. (Eds.): *Psychotropic Drugs.* Amsterdam, Elsevier, 1957, pp. 262-672.

Chiocchio, S.R., Biscardi, A.M. and Tramezzani, J.H.: Catecholamines in the carotid body of the cat. *Nature* (London), *141:* 183-192, 1966.

Christensen, K.: *Venous System in Blood Vessels and Lymphatics,* ed. by D.S. Abramson, New York, Academic Press, 1962, pp. 192-196.

Colburn, R.W., Goodwin, F.K., Murphy, D.L., Bunney, W.E. and Davis, J.M.: Quantitative studies of norepinephrine uptake by synaptosomes. *Biochem Pharmacol, 17:* 957-964, 1968.

Crane, R.K.: Na+-dependent transport in the intestine and other animal tissue. *Fed Proc, 24:* 1000-1006, 1965.

Crout, J.R.: Effect of inhibiting both catechol-O-methyl transferase and monoamine oxidase on cardiovascular responses to norepinephrine. *Proc Soc Exp Biol Med* (N.Y.), *108:* 482-484, 1961.

Crout, J.R.: Catecholamines metabolism in pheochromocytoma and essential hypertension. In: Manger, W. M. (Ed.): *Hormones and Hypertension.* Springfield, Thomas, 1966, pp. 3-40.

Crout, J.R. and Alpers, H.S., Tatum, E.L. and Shore, P.A.: Release of Metaraminol (aramine) from the heart by sympathetic nerve stimulation. *Science, 145:* 828-829, 1964.

Crout, R. and Shore, P.A.: Release of metaraminol (aramine) from the heart by sympathetic nerve stimulation. *Clin Res, 12:* 180, 1964.

Cullingham, B.A. and Mann, M.: Depletion and replacement of the adrenaline and noradrenaline contents of the rat adrenal gland following treatment with reserpine. *Br J Pharmacol, 18:* 138-149, 1962.

Dahlström, A.: The effect of reserpine and tetrabenazine on the accumulation of noradrenaline in the rat sciatic nerve after ligation. *Acta Physiol Scand, 69:* 167-169, 1967.

Dahlström, A. and Häggendal, J.: Some quantitative studies on the noradrenaline content in the cell bodies and terminals of a sympathetic adrenergic neuron system. *Acta Physiol Scand, 67:* 271-277, 1966a.

Dahlström, A. and Häggendal, J.: Studies on the transport and life span of amine storage granules in a peripheral adrenergic neuron system. *Acta Physiol Scand, 67:* 278-288, 1966b.

Dairman, W., Gordon, R., Spector, S., Sjoerdsma, A. and Udenfriend, S.: Increased synthesis of catecholamines in the intact rat following administration of α-adrenergic blocking agents. *Mol Pharmacol, 4:* 457-464, 1968.

Dale, H.H.: On some physiological actions of ergot. *J Physiol* (London), *34:* 163-206, 1906.

Davis, J.O.: The mechanisms of salt and water retention in cardiac failure. *Hosp Prac,* 5 (10) : 63-76, 1970.

Day, M.D. and Rand, M.J.: Some observations of α-methyl-dopa. *Br J Pharmacol, 22:* 72-86, 1964.

Dawson, J. and Bone, A.: The relationship between urine volume and urinary adrenalin and noradrenalin excretion in a group of psychotic patients. *Brit J Psychiat, 109:* 629-630, 1963.

Dean, C.R. and Hope, D.B.: The isolation of neurophysin-I and -II from bovine pituitary neurosecretory granules separated on a large scale from other subcellular organelles. Demonstration on slow equalibration of neurosecretory granules during centrifugation in a sucrose density gradient. *Biochem J, 106:* 565-573, 1968.

DeChamplain, J. and van Ameringen, M.R.: Regulation of blood pressure by sympathetic nerve fibers and adrenal medulla in normotensive and hypertensive rats. *Circ Res, 31:* 617-628, 1972.

DeChamplain, J., Mueller, R.A. and Axelrod, J.: Turnover and synthesis of norepinephrine in experimental hypertension in rats. *Circ Res, 25:* 285-292, 1969.

De LaLande, I.S. and Waterson, J.G.: Site of action of cocaine on the perfused artery. *Nature* (London), *214:* 313-314, 1967.

Dengler, H.J., Spiegel, H.E. and Titus, E.O.: Effects of drugs on uptake of isotopic norepinephrine by cat tissues. *Nature* (London), *191:* 816-817, 1961.

Dengler, H.J., Michaelson, I.H., Spiegel, H.E. and Titus, E.O.: The uptake of labeled norepinephrine by isolated brain and other tissues of the cat. *Int J Neuropharmacol, 1:* 23-38, 1962.

DeQuattro, V., Nagatsu, T., Maronde, R. and Alexander, N.: Catecholamine synthesis in rabbits with neurogenic hypertension. *Circ Res, 24:* 545-555, 1969.

DeRobertis, E. and Ferreira, A. Vaz: Electron microscope study of the excretion of catechol-containing droplets in the adrenal medulla. *Exp Cell Res, 12:* 568-574, 1957.

DeSchaepdryver, A.F. and Leroy, J.G.: Urine volume and catecholamine excretion in man. *Acta Cardiol* (Brux.) , *16:* 631-638, 1961.

Doyle, A.E. and Smirk, F.H.: The neurogenic component in hypertension. *Circulation, 12:* 543-552, 1955.

Draskóczy, P.R. and Trendelenburg, U.: The uptake of l- and d-norepinephrine by the isolated perfused rabbit heart in relation to the stereospecificity of the sensitizing action of cocaine. *J Pharmacol Exp Ther, 156:* 109-113, 1968.

Draskóczy, P.R. and Trendelenburg, U.: Intraneuronal and extraneuronal accumulation of sympathomimetic amines in the isolated nictitating membrane of the cat. *J Pharmacol Exp Ther, 174:* 290-306, 1970.

Douglas, W.W. and Rubin, R.P.: The mechanism of catecholamine release from the adrenal medulla and the role of calcium in stimulus-secretion coupling. *J Physiol* (London) , *167:* 288-310, 1963.

Dunham, E.W. and Zimmerman, B.A.: Release of prostaglandin-like material from dog kidney during nerve stimulation. *Am J Physiol, 219:* 1279-1285, 1970.

Dunlop, D. and Shanks, R.G.: Selective blockade of adrenoceptive beta receptors in the heart. *Br J Pharmacol, 32:* 201-218, 1968.

Eade, N.R.: The distribution of the catecholamines in homogenates of the bovine adrenal medulla. *J Physiol* (London) , *141:* 183-192, 1958.

Ehringer, B. and Sporrong, B.: Neuronal and extraneuronal localisation of noradrenaline in the rat heart after perfusion at high concentration. *Experientia, 24:* 265-266, 1968.

Eiff, A.W. von: The role of the autonomic nerves system in the etiology and pathogenesis of essential hypertension. *Jap Circ J, 34:* 147-153, 1970.

Eisenfeld, A.J., Axelrod, J. and Krakoff, L.: Inhibition of the extraneuronal accumulation and metabolism of norepinephrine by adrenergic blocking agents. *J Pharmacol Exp Ther, 156:* 107-113, 1967a.

Eisenfeld, A.J., Landsberg, L. and Axelrod, J.: Effect of drugs on the accumulation and metabolism of extraneuronal norepinephrine in the rat heart. *J Pharmacol Exp Ther, 158:* 378-385, 1967b.

Elliott, T.R.: The action of adrenalin. *J Physiol* (London), *32:* 401-467, 1905.

Engelman, K. and Portnoy, B.: A sensitive double-isotope derivative assay for norepinephrine: Normal resting human plasma levels. *Circ Res, 26:* 53-57, 1970.

Engelman, K., Portnoy, B. and Sjoerdsma, A.: Plasma catecholamine concentrations in patients with hypertension. *Circ Res* (Supplement), *1:* 26-27, 1970.

Engelman, K. and Sjoerdsma, A.: A new test for pheochromocytoma: pressor responsiveness to tyramine. *JAMA, 61:* 229-241, 1964.

Engelman, K. and Sjoerdsma, A.: The adrenal medulla: catecholamines and pheochromocytoma. In: *Clinician-1, The Adrenal Gland,* 1971, p. 111-125.

Euler, U.S. von: Zur kenntnis der pharmakologischen wirkungen von nativsekreten und extrackten mannlicher accessorischer ceschechtdrusen. *Arch Exp Path Pharmakol, 175:* 78-, 1934.

Euler, U.S. von: Identification of the sympathomimetic ergone in adrenergic nerves of cattle (Sympathin-N) with Laevo-Noradrenaline. *Acta Physiol Scand, 16:* 63-74, 1948.

Euler, U.S. von and Lishajko, F.: Dopamine in mammalian lung and spleen. *Acta Physiol Pharmacol Neerl, 6:* 295-303, 1957.

Falck, B., Hillarp, N.A. and Torp, A.: A new type of chromaffin cells, probably storing dopamine. *Nature* (London), *183:* 267-268, 1959.

Falck, B.: Observation on the possibilities of the cellular localization of monoamines by a fluorescence method. *Acta Physiol Scand, 56,* Supplement, *197:* 6-25, 1962.

Farmer, J.B., and Campbell, I.K.: Calcium and magnesium ions: influence of response of an isolated artery to sympathetic nerve stimulation, noradrenaline and tyramine. *Br J Pharmacol, 29:* 319-328, 1967.

Farnebo, L.O. and Malmfors, T.: Histochemical studies on the uptake of noradrenaline and α-methyl-noradrenaline in the perfused rat heart. *Eur J Pharmacol, 5:* 313-320, 1969.

Farnebo, L. and Hamberger, B.: Release of norepinephrine from isolated rat iris by field stimulation. *J Pharmacol Exp Ther, 172:* 332-341, 1970.

Feldberg, W. and Lewis, G.P.: The action of peptides on the adrenal medulla. Release of adrenaline by bradykinin and angiotensin. *J Physiol* (London), *171:* 98-108, 1964.

Finkielman, S., Worcel, M. and Agrest, A.: Hemodynamic patterns in essential hypertension. *Circulation, 21:* 356-368, 1965.

Fischer, J.E., Mussacchio, J., Kopin, I.J. and Axelrod, J.: Effect of denervation on the uptake and β-hydroxylation of tyramine in the rat salivary gland. *Life Sci, 3:* 413-419, 1964.

Fischer, J., Kopin, I. and Axelrod, J.: Evidence for extraneuronal binding of norepinephrine. *J Pharmacol Exp Ther, 147:* 181-185, 1965.

Folkow, B.: Description of the myogenic hypothesis. *Circ Res* 14-15 Supplement, 1, 279-287, 1964.

Folkow, B., Haggendal, J. and Lisander, B.: Extent of release and elimination of noradrenaline at peripheral adrenergic nerve terminals. *Acta Physiol Scand* (Supplement), *307:* 1-38, 1967.

Frohlich, E.D., Tarazi, R.C. and Dustan, H.P.: Re-examination of the hemodynamics of hypertension. *Am J Med Sci, 257:* 9-21, 1969.

Fujimoto, S. and Lockett, M.F.: The diuretic actions of prostaglandin E. and of noradrenaline, and the occurence of a prostaglandin E_1-like substance in the renal lymph of cats. *Physiol* (London) , *208:* 1-19, 1970.

Fuxe, K.: The distribution of monoamine nerve terminals in the central nervous system. *Acta Physiol Scand* (Supplment 247) , *64:* 37-85, 1965.

Giachetti, A. and Shore, P.A.: Studies *in vitro* of amine uptake mechanisms in heart. *Biochem Pharmacol, 15:* 607-614, 1966.

Gifford, Ray W., Jr.: Renovascular hypertension. *Postgrad Med, 52* (3) : 110-116, 1972.

Gillespie, J.S. and Hamilton, D.N.H.: A possible active transport of noradrenaline into arterial smooth muscle cells. *J Physiol* (London) , *181:* 69, 1965.

Gillis, C.N. and Paton, D.M.: Cation dependence of sympathetic transmitter retention by slices of rat ventricle. *Br J Pharmacol, 29:* 309-318, 1967.

Gitlow, S.E., Mendlowitz, M., Wilk, E.K., Wilk, S., Wolf, R.L. and Naftchi, N.E.: Plasma clearance of dl-β-H^3-norepinephrine in normal human subjects and patients with essential hypertension. *J Clin Invest, 43:* 2009-2015, 1964.

Gitlow, S.E., Mendlowitz, M., Bertani, L.M., Wilk, E.K. and Glabman, S.: Tritium excretion of normotensive and hypertensive subjects after administration of tritiated norepinephrine. *J Lab Clin Med, 73:* 129-134, 1969.

Glynn, I.M.: The action of cardiac glycosides on ion movements. *Pharmac Rev, 16:* 381-407, 1964.

Goodall, McCh.: Hydroxytyramine in mammalian heart. *Nature* (London) , *166:* 738, 1950.

Goodall, McCh.: Studies of adrenaline and noradrenaline in mammalian heart and suprarenals. *Acta Physiol Scand,* (Supplement 85) , *24:* 1-51, 1951.

Gordon, R., Reid, J.V.O., Sjoerdsma, A. and Udenfriend, S.: Increased synthesis of norepinephrine in the rat heart on electrical stimulation of the stellate ganglia. *Mol Pharmacol, 2:,* 610-613, 1966a.

Gordon, R., Spector, S., Sjoerdsma, A. and Udenfriend, S.: Increased synthesis of norepinephrine in the intact rat during exercise and exposure to cold. *J Pharmacol Exp Ther, 153:* 440-447, 1966b.

Govier, W.C.: Myocardial alpha adrenergic receptors and their role in the production of a positive inotropic effect by sympathomimetic amines. *J Pharmacol Exp Ther, 159:* 82-90, 1968.

Green, A.F.: Antihypertensive Drugs. In Garattini, S., and Shore, P.A. (Eds.) : *Advances in Pharmacology.* New York, Academic Press, 1962, vol. I.

Green, R.D. and Miller, J.W.: Evidence for the active transport of epinephrine and norepinephrine by the uterus of the rat. *J Pharmacol Exp Ther, 152:* 42-50, 1966.

Hathaway, P.W., Brehm, M.L., Clapp, J.R. and Bogdonoff, M.D.: Urine flow, catecholamines, and blood pressure. *Psychosom Med, 31:* 20-30, 1969.

Hertting, G., Axelrod, J. and Patrick, R.W.: Action of bretylium and guanethidine on the uptake and release of ^{3}H-noradrenaline. *Br J Pharmacol, 18:* 161-166, 1962a.

Hertting, G., Axelrod, J. and Whitby, L.G.: Effect of drugs on the uptake and metabolism of ^{3}H-norepinephrine. *J Pharmacol Exp Ther, 134:* 145-153, 1961.

Hertting, G., Axelrod, J., Kopin, I.J. and Whitby, L.G.: Lack of uptake of catecholamines after chronic denervation of sympathetic nerves. *Nature* (London) , *189:* 66, 1961b.

Hertting, G., Potter, L.T. and Axelrod, J.: Effect of decentralization and ganglionic blocking agents on the spontaneous release of ^{3}H-norepinephrine. *J Pharmacol Exp Ther 135:* 289-292, 1962b.

Higgins, C.B., Vatner, S.F., Franklin, D. and Braunwald, E.: Effects of prostaglandin A, (PGA) on left ventricular dynamics in conscious dogs. *Clin Res 19:* 350, 1971.

Hillarp, N.A.: Structure of the synapse and the peripheral innervation apparatus of autonomic nervous system. *Acta Anat 2,* (Supplement) , *4:* 1-153, 1946.

Hillarp, N.A.: Further observation on the state of catecholamines in the adrenal medullary granules. *Acta Physiol Scand, 47:* 271-279, 1959.

Hirano, I.: Studies on hemodynamics in essential hypertension—with special reference to the correlation with sympathetic nervous system. *Sapporo Med J, 36:* 159-171, 1969.

Hoobler, S.W., Agrest, A. and Warzynski, R.J.: Biochemical determination of blood and urine catecholamines as a measure of sympathoadrenal activity in hypertension. *J Clin Invest, 33:* 943-944, 1954.

Hornykiewicz, O.: Dopamine (3-hydroxytyramine) and brain function. *Pharmac Rev, 18:* 925-964, 1966.

Horton, E.W.: Hypotheses on physiological roles of prostaglandins. *Physiol Rev, 49:* 122-161, 1969.

Ikeda, M., Levitt, M. and Udenfriend, S.: Hydroxylation of phenylalanine by purified preparations of adrenal and brain tyrosine hydroxylase. *Biochem Biophys Res Commun, 18:* 482-488, 1965.

Ikoma, T.: Studies on catechols with reference to hypertension. *Jap Circ J, 29:* 1269-1286, 1965.

Iversen, L.L.: The uptake of noradrenalin by the isolated perfused rat heart. *Br J Pharmacol, 21:* 523-537, 1963 .

Iversen, L.L.: The uptake of catecholamines at high perfusion concentrations in the rat isolated heart; a novel catecholamine uptake process. *Br J Pharmacol, 25:* 18-33, 1965.

Iversen, L.L. and Kravitz, E.A.: Sodium dependence of transmitter uptake at adrenergic nerve terminals. *Mol Pharmacol, 2:* 360-362, 1966.

Iversen, L.L., Glowinski, J., and Axelrod, J.: The uptake and storage of ^{3}H-norepinephrine in the reserpine-pretreated rat heart. *J Pharmacol Exp Ther, 150:* 173-178, 1965.

Iversen, L.L., Glowinski, J. and Axelrod, J.: The physiological disposition and metabolism of norepinephrine in immunosympathectomized animals. *J Pharmacol Exp Ther, 151:* 273-284, 1966.

Iyer, N.T., McGeer, P.L. and McGeer, E.G.: Conversion of tyrosine to catecholamines by rat brain slices. *Canad J Biochem Physiol, 41:* 1565-1570, 1963.

Johns, V.J. and Brunjes, S.: Pheochromocytoma. *Am J Cardiol, 9:* 120-125, 1962.

Jonsson, G.: Microfluorimetric studies on the formaldehyde-induced fluorescence of noradrenaline in adrenergic nerves of rat iris. *J Histochem Cytochem, 17:* 714-723, 1969.

Jonsson, G. and Sachs, C.: Subcellular distribution of ^{3}H-noradrenaline in adrenergic nerves of mouse atrium—effect of reserpine, monoamine oxidase and tyrosine hydroxylase inhibition. *Acta Physiol Scand, 80:* 307-322, 1970.

Jonsson, G., Hamberger, B., Malmfors, T. and Sachs, C.: Uptake and accumulation of ^{3}H-noradrenaline in adrenergic nerves of rat iris. Effect of reserpine, monoamine oxidase and tyrosine hydroxylase inhibition. *Europ J Pharmacol, 8:* 58-72, 1969.

Kalsner, S. and Nickerson, M.: The disposition of norepinephrine and epinephrine in vascular tissue, determined by the technique of oil immersion. *J Pharmacol Exp Ther, 165:* 152-165, 1969.

Keswani, G., D'Iorio, A. and Fitt, E.: The influence of sulfhydryl on the storage release of catecholamines in the isolated chromaffin granules of the ox adrenal medulla. *Arch Int Pharmacodyn, 181:* 57-67, 1969.

Kipnis, D.M. and Parrish, J.E.: Role of Na$^+$ and K$^+$ on sugar (2-deoxyglucose) and amino acid α-amino-isobutyric acid) transport in striated muscle. *Fed Proc, 24:* 1051-1059, 1965.

Kirschner, N.: Storage and secretion of adrenal catecholamines. In Costa, E., and Greengrad, P. (Eds.): *Advances in Biochemical Psychopharmacology*. New York, Raven Press, 1969, vol. 1, pp. 7171-89.

Kopin, I.J.: Storage and metabolism of catecholamines: the role of monoamine oxidase. *Pharmac Rev, 16:* 179-191, 1964.

Kopin, I.J. and Gorden, E.K.: Metabolism of norepinephrine - H³ released by tyramine and reserpine. *J Pharmacol Exp Ther, 138:* 351-359, 1962.

Kopin, I.J. and Gorden, E.K.: Metabolism of administered and drug-released norepinephrine - 7 - H³ in the rat. *J Pharmacol Exp Ther, 140:* 207-216, 1963.

Kopin, I.J., Fischer, J.E., Musacchio, J.M. and Horst, W.D.: Evidence for a false neurochemical transmitter as a mechanism for the hypotensive effect of monoamine oxidase inhibitors. *Proc Nat Acad Sci* (Wash.) , *52:* 716-721, 1964.

Kopin, I.J., Fischer, J.E., Musacchio, J.M., Horst, W.D. and Weise, V.K.: False neurochemical transmitters and the mechanism of sympathetic blockade by monoamine oxidase inhibitors. *J Pharmacol Exp Ther, 147:* 186-193, 1965.

Kopin, I.J., Weise, U.K. and Sedvall, G.: Effect of false transmitters on norepinephrine synthesis. *J Pharmacol Exp Ther, 170:* 246-252, 1969.

Kopin, I.J.: Biochemical aspects of release of norepinephrine and other amines from sympathetic nerve endings. *Pharmacol Rev, 18:* 513-523, 1966.

Krakoff, L.F., DeChamplain, J. and Axelrod, J.: Abnormal storage of norepinephrine in experimental hypertension in the rat. *Circ Res, 21:* 583-591, 1967.

Kuriyama, H.: Effect of calcium and magnesium on neuromuscular transmission in the hypogastric nerve vas deferens preparation of the guinea-pig. *J Physiol* (London) , *175:* 211-230, 1964.

Lands, A.M. and Brown, J.G., Jr.: A comparison of the cardiac stimulating and bronchodilator action of selected sympathomimetic amines. *Proc Soc Exp Biol Med, 116:* 331-333, 1964.

Lands, A.M., Luduena, F.P. and Buzzo, H.J.: Differentiation of receptors responsive to isoproterenol. *Life Sci, 6:* 2241, 1967.

Langley, J.N.: On reaction of cells and of nerve endings on certain poisons, chiefly as regards reaction of striated muscle to nicotine and to curare. *J Physiol* (London) , *33:* 374-413, 1905.

Lee, J.B., McGiff, J.C., Kannegiesser, H., Aykent, Y.Y., Mudd, J.G. and Frawley, T.F.: Prostaglandin A,: Antihypertensive and renal effects. *Ann Intern Med, 74:* 703-710, 1971.

Levin, E.Y. and Kaufman, S.: Studies on the enzyme catalysing the conversion of 3,4-dihydroxyphenylethyl-amine to norepinephrine. *J Biol Chem, 236:* 2043-2044, 1961.

Levin, J.A. and Furchgott, R.F.: Interactions between potentiating agents of adrenergic amines in rabbit aortic strips. *J Pharmacol Exp Ther, 172:* 320-331, 1970.

Levitt, M., Spector, S., Sjoerdsma, A. and Udenfriend, S.: Elucidation of the rate-limiting step in norepinephrine biosynthesis in the perfused guinea-pig heart. *J Pharmacol Exp Ther, 148:* 1-8, 1965.

Levy, B.: A comparison of the adrenergic receptor blocking properties of 1- (4'-methylphenyl) -2-isopropylamino-propanol HCl and propranolol. *J Pharmacol Exp Ther, 156:* 452-462, 1967.

Levy, B.: Alterations of adrenergic responses by N-isopropyl methoxamine. *J Pharmacol Exp Ther, 146:* 129-138, 1964.

Levy, B.: The adrenergic blocking activity of N-tert-butylmethoxamine (butoxamine). *J Pharmacol Exp Ther, 151:* 413-422, 1966a.

Levy, B.: Dimethyl isopropylmethoxamine: a selective beta receptor blocking agent. *Br J Pharmacol, 27:* 277-285, 1966b.

Lightman, S.L. and Iversen, L.L.: The role of uptake$_2$ in the extraneuronal metabolism of catecholamines in the isolated rat heart. *Brit J Pharmacol, 37:* 639-649, 1969.

Lindmar, R. and Muscholl, E.: Die Wirkung von pharmaka auf die elimination von noradrenal aus der perfusion sflussigkeit und die noradrenalin aufnahme in das isolierte herz. *Arch Exp Path Pharmak, 247:* 469-492, 1964.

Lishajko, F.: Release, reuptake and net uptake of dopamine, noradrenaline and adrenaline in isolated sheep adrenal medullary granules. *Acta Physiol Scand, 76:* 159-171, 1969.

Lishajko, F.: Dopamine secretion from the isolated perfused sheep adrenal. *Acta Physiol Scand, 76:* 159-171, 1970a.

Lishajko, F.: Release and uptake of dopamine in isolated granules from a human carotid body tumor. *Acta Physiol Scand, 79:* 533-536, 1970b.

Loewi, O.: Uber humorale Ubertragbarkeit der Herznervenwirkung I. Mitteilung. *Pflugers Arch Ges Physiol, 189:* 239-242, 1921.

Louis, W.J.: Turnover of catecholamines in experimental hypertension. *Circ Res* (Supplement 2) , *26-27:* 49-53, 1970.

Lucchesi, B.R. and Whitsitt, L.S.: The pharmacology of Beta-Adrenergic blocking agents. *Prog Cardiovas Dis, 11:* 410-430, 1969.

Malindzak, Jr., Van Dyke, A.H., Green, H.D. and Meredith, J.H.: Alpha and Beta adrenergic receptors in the coronary vascular bed. *Arch Int Pharmacodyn, 197:* 112-122, 1972.

Malmfors, T.: Fluorescent histo-chemical studies on the uptake and storage and release of catecholamine. *Circ Res* (suppl. 3) , *20-21:* 25-42, 1967.

Manger, W.M.: Observations on plasma catecholamines in patients with diastolic hypertension. *Am J Cardiol, 9:* 731-742, 1962.

Maxwell, R.A., Wastila, W.B. and Eckhardt, S.B.: Some factors determining the response of rabbit aortic strips to dl-norepinephrine-7-³H hydrochloride and the influence of cocaine, guanethidine and methylphenidate on these factors. *J Pharmacol Exp Ther, 151:* 253-261, 1966.

Maxwell, R.A., Eckhardt, S.B. and Wastila, W.B.: Concerning the distribution of endogenous norepinephrine in the adventitial and media-intimal layers of the rabbit aorta and the capacity of these layers to bind tritiated norepinephrine. *J Pharmacol Exp Ther, 161:* 34-39, 1968.

McCubbin, J. and Page, I.H.: Renal pressor system and neurogenic control of arterial pressure. *Circ Res, 12:* 553-559, 1963.

McGeer, P.L., Bagchi, S.P. and McGeer, E.G.: Subcellular localization of tyrosine hydroxylase in beef caudate nucleus. *Life Sci, 4:* 1859-1867, 1965.

McGiff, J.C., Crowshaw, K., Terragno, N.A. and Lonigro, A.J.: Release of a prostaglandin-like substance into renal venous blood in response to angiotensin II. *Circ Res* (Supplement 1) , *26-27:* 121-129, 1970.

Melmon, K. L.: Catecholamines and the adrenal medulla. In: Williams, R.H. (Ed.) *Textbook of Endocrinology,* 4th ed., Philadelphia, Saunders, 1968, pp. 379-403.

Montagu, K.A.: Catechol compounds in rat tissues and in brains of different animals. *Nature* (London) , *180:* 244-245, 1957.

Mueller, R.A., Thoenen, H. and Axelrod, J.: Increase in tyrosine hydroxylase activity after reserpine administration. *J Pharmacol Exp Ther, 169:* 74-79, 1969a.

Mueller, R.A., Thoenen, H. and Axelrod, J.: Inhibition of transsynaptically increased tyrosine hydroxylase activity by cyclohexamide and actinomycin D. *Mal Pharmacol, 5:* 463-469, 1969b.

Mussacchio, J.M.: Subcellular distribution of adrenal tyrosine hydroxylase. *Biochem Pharmacol, 17:* 1470-1473, 1968.

Nagatsu, T., Levitt, M. and Udenfriend, S.: Tyrosine hydroxylase, the initial step in norepinephrine biosynthesis. *J Biol Chem, 239:* 2910-2917, 1964.

Nakano, J.: Prostaglandins and the circulation. *Mod Concepts Cardiovasc Dis, 40* (10) : 49-54, 1971.

Neff, N.H. and Costa, E.: The influence of monoamine oxidase inhibitor on catecholamine synthesis. *Life Sci, 5:* 951-959, 1966.

Nestel, P.J.: Blood pressure and catecholamine excretion after mental stress in labile hypertension, *Circ Res* (Supplement 2), *26-27:* 75-81, 1970.

Nestel, P.J. and Doyle, A.E.: Excretion of free noradrenaline and adrenaline by healthy young subjects and by patients with essential hypertension. *Australas Ann Med, 17:* 295-299, 1968.

Nestel, P.J., F.R.A.C.P. and Esler, M.D.: Patterns of catecholamine excretion in urine in hypertension. *Circ Res* (Suppl. 2), *26-27:* 75-81, 1970.

Ngai, S.H., Neff, N.H. and Costa, E.: Effect of pargyline on the rate of conversion of tyrosine[14]C to norepinephrine[14]C. *Life Sci, 7:* 847-855, 1968.

Norberg, K.A. and Hamberger, B.: The sympathetic adrenergic neuron. Some characteristics revealed by histochemical studies on the intraneuronal distribution of the transmitter. *Acta Physiol Scand* (Supplement 238), *63:* 1-42, 1964.

Oberg, B. and Rosell, S.: Sympathetic control of consecutive vascular sections in canine subcutaneous adipose tissue. *Acta Physiol Scand, 71:* 47-56, 1967.

Oliver, G. and Schafer, E.A.: The physiological effects of extracts of the suprarenal capsules. *J Physiol* (London), *18:* 230-276, 1895.

Oliverio, A. and Stjärne, L.: Acceleration of noradrenaline turnover in the mouse heart by cold exposure. *Life Sci, 4:* 2339-2343, 1965.

Overy, H.R., Pfister, R. and Chidsey, C.A.: Studies on the renal excretion of norepinephrine. *J Clin Invest, 46:* 482-489, 1967.

Pappas, G.D. and Bennett, M.V.: Specialized junctions involved in electrical transmission between neurons. *Ann NY Acad Sci, 137:* 495-508, 1966.

Paton, D.M.: Cation and metabolic requirement for retention of metaraminol by rat uterine horns. *Br J Pharmacol, 33:* 277-286, 1968.

Peach, M.J., Bumpus, F.M. and Khairallah, P.A.: Inhibition of norepinephrine uptake in hearts by angiotensin II and analogs. *J Pharmacol Exp Ther, 167:* 291-299, 1969.

Peart, W.S.: The nature of splenic sympathin. *J Physiol* (London), *108:* 491-501, 1949.

Pease, D.C.: *Microscopic and Submicroscopic Anatomy. Blood Vessels and Lymphatics,* D.I. Abramson, (Ed.), New York, Academic Press, 1962, pp. 12-25.

Potter, L.T. and Axelrod, J.: Subcellular localization of catecholamines in tissues of the rat. *J Pharmacol Exp Ther, 142:* 291-298, 1963a.

Potter, L.T. and Axelrod, J.: Properties of norepinephrine storage particles of the rat heart. *J Pharmacol Exp Ther, 142:* 299-305, 1963b.

Robinson, R.L.: Stimulation of the catecholamine output of the isolated perfused adrenal gland of the dog by angiotensin and Bradykinin. *J Pharmacol Exp Ther, 156:* 252-257, 1967.

Roth, R.H.: Action of angiotensin on adrenergic nerve endings: enhancement of norepinephrine biosynthesis. *Fed Proc, 31:* 1358-1364, 1972.

Rubin, R.P. and Miele, E.: A study of the differential secretion of epinephrine and norepinephrine from the perfused cat adrenal gland. *J Pharmacol Exp Ther, 164:* 115-121, 1968.

Rutledge, C.P. and Weiner, N.: The effect of reserpine upon the synthesis of norepinephrine in the isolated rabbit heart. *J Pharmacol Exp Ther, 157:* 290-302, 1967.

Sano, I., Gamo, T., Kakimoto, Y., Taniguchi, K., Takesada, M. and Nishinuma, K.: Distribution of catechol compounds in human brain. *Biochem Biophys Acat, 32:* 586, 57, 1959.

Sedvall, G.C. and Kopin, I.J.: Acceleration of norepinephrine synthesis in the rat submaxillary gland *in vivo* during sympathetic nerve stimulation. *Life Sci, 6:* 45-52, 1967a.

Sedvall, G.C. and Kopin, I.J.: Influence of sympathetic denervation and nerve impulse activity of tyrosine hydroxylase in the rat submaxillary gland. *Biochem Pharmacol, 16:* 39-46, 1967b.

Shore, P.A., Busfield, D. and Alpers, H.S.: Binding and release of metaraminol: mechanism of norepinephrine depletion by α-methyl-m-tyrosine and related agents. *J Pharmacol Exp Ther, 146:* 194-199, 1964.

Slotkin, T.A. and Krishner, N.: Uptake, storage and distribution of amines in bovine adrenal medullary vesicles. *Mol Pharmacol, 7:* 581-592, 1971.

Smith, A.D.: *Biochemistry of Adrenal Chromaffin Granules. The Interaction of Drugs and Subcellular Components on Animal Cells.* P.N. Campbell, (ed.), J. and A. Churchill Ltd. (London), 1968, pp. 239-292.

Somova, L. and Dochev, D.: Changes in the renin activity in rats with experimental hypertension treated with (prostaglandins) PGE and PGE$_2$. *Dokl Bolg Akad Nauk, 23:* 1581-1584, 1970.

Stjärne, L., Roth, R.H., Bloom, F.E. and Giarman, N.J.: Norepinephrine concentrating mechanisms in sympathetic nerve trunks. *J Pharmacol Exp Ther, 171:* 70-79, 1970.

Sugrue, M.F. and Shore, P.A.: The mode of sodium dependency of the adrenergic neuron amine carrier. Evidence for a second, sodium-dependent, optically specific and reserpine-sensitive system. *J Pharmacol Exp Ther, 170:* 239-245, 1970.

Taugner, G. and Hasselbach, W.: Die Bedeutung der sulfhydryl-Gruppen fruden catecholamin-Transport der vesikel des neuennierenmarbes. *Naunyn Schmiedeberg Arch Pharm Exp Path, 260:* 58-79, 1968.

Thoenen, H., Mueller, R.A. and Axelrod, J.: Increased tyrosine hydroxylase activity after drug induced alteration of sympathetic transmission. *Nature* (London), *221:* 1264, 1969a.

Thoenen, H., Mueller, R.A. and Axelrod, J.: Trans-synaptic induction of adrenal tyrosine hydroxylase. *J Pharmacol Exp Ther, 169:* 249-254, 1969b.

Thoenen, H. and Tranzer, J.P.: Zur Moglichkeit der chemischen Sympathektomie durch selektive Zerstorung adrenerger Nervenendegungen mit 6-Hydroxydopamin (6-OH-DA). *Naunyn Schmiedebergs Arch Pharmac Exp Path, 260:* 212-213, 1968a.

Thoenen, H. and Tranzer, J.P.: Chemical sympathectomy by selective destruction of adrenergic nerve endings with 6-hydroxydopamine. *Naunyn Schmiedebergs Arch Pharmac Exp Path, 261:* 271-288, 1968b.

Tranzer, J.P. and Thoenen, H.: Ultramorphologische Veranderungen der sympathischen Nervendegungen der Katze nach Vorke handlung mit 5- und 6-Hydroxy-Dopamin. *Naunyn Schmiedebergs Arch Pharmac exp Path, 257:* 343-344, 1967.

Tranzer, J.P. and Thoenen, H.: An electron microscopic study of selective, acute degeneration of sympathetic nerve terminals after administration of 6-hydroxydopamine. *Experientia, 24:* 155-156, 1968.

Trendelenburg, U.: Supersensitivity by cocaine to dextrorotatory isomers of norepinephrine and epinephrine. *J Pharmacol Exp Ther, 148:* 329-338, 1965.

Trendelenburg, U.: Mechanisms of supersensitivity and subsensitivity to sympathomimetic amines. *Pharmacol Rev, 18:* 629-640, 1966.

Trendelenburg, U., Draskóczy, P.R. and Pluchino, S.: The density of adrenergic innervation of the cat's nictitating membrane as a factor influencing the sensitivity of the isolated preparation to L-norepinephrine. *J Pharmacol Exp Ther, 166:* 14-25, 1969.

Udenfriend, S., Zaltzman-Nirenberg, P.: On the mechanism of the norepinephrine release produced by alpha-methyl-meta-tyrosine. *J Pharmacol Exp Ther, 138:* 196-199, 1962.

Vane, J.R.: The release and fate of vasoactive hormones in the circulation. *Br J Pharmacol, 35:* 209-242, 1969.

Van Woert, M.H. and Korb, F.: Effect of whole-body x-irradiation on tyrosine hydroxylase and catecholamine levels. *Life Sci, 9:* 227-232, 1970.

Wakade, A.R. and Furchgott, R.F.: Metabolic requirements for the uptake and storage of norepinephrine by the isolated left atrium of the guinea-pig. *J Pharmacol Exp Ther, 163:* 123-135, 1968.

Whittaker, V.P.: Some properties of synaptic membrane isolated from the central nervous system. *Ann NY Acad Sci, 137:* 982-998, 1966.

Whitby, L.G., Hertting, G. and Axelrod, J.: The fate of H³-norepinephrine in animals. *J Pharmacol Exp Ther, 132:* 193-201, 1961.

Weiner, W. and Alousi, A.: Influence of nerve stimulation on rate of synthesis of norepinephrine. *Fed Proc, 25:* 396, 1966.

Weiner, N., Perkins, M. and Sidman, R.L.: Effect of reserpine on noradrenaline content of innervated and denervated brown adipose tissue of the rat. *Nature* (London), *193:* 137-138, 1962.

Weiner, N. and Rabadjija, M.: Effect of nerve stimulation on synthesis of norepinephrine from tyrosine during and after the stimulation period. *Fed Proc, 27:* 240, 1968a.

Weiner, N. and Rabadjija, M.: The effect of nerve stimulation on the synthesis and metabolism of norepinephrine in the isolated guinea-pig hypogastric nerve-vas deferens preparations. *J Pharmacol Exp Ther, 160:* 61-71, 1968b.

Weiner, N. and Rabadjija, M.: The regulation of norepinephrine synthesis. Effect of puromycin on the accelerated synthesis of norepinephrine associated with nerve stimulation. *J Pharmacol Exp Ther, 164:* 103-114, 1968c.

Wurtman, R.J. and Axelrod, J.: Control of the enzymatic synthesis of adrenaline in the adrenal medulla by adrenal cortical steroid. *J Biol Chem, 241:* 2301-2305, 1966.

Zimmerman, B.G., Gomer, S.K. and Lio, J.C.: Action of angiotensin on vascular adrenergic nerve endings: facilitation or norepinephrine release. *Fed Proc, 31:* 1344-1350, 1972.

INDEX

A

Adrenal vesicles, 10
  composition and function of, 11
  mechanism of release, 10
Adrenergic neuron, 6-8
Adrenergic receptors, 108-117
  classification, 109, 110
  complications of blockade of beta, 117
  definition, 111
  physiological significance of beta, 114-115
  response of circulatory system to stimulation
    of, 112
  result of blockade of cardiac, 113
  specificity of drugs blocking beta, 110
  usefulness of blockade of beta, 116
Angiotensin, 98, 132
  action/effect on adrenal
    cortex and aldosterone secretion, 100, 101,
      132
    adrenal medulla, 100
    autonomic nervous system, 100
    cardiovascular system, 99
  formation and inactivation, 98, 99, 132
Antihypertensive agents pharmacology of, 163-
  184
  alpha-methyldopa, 34, 169
    accumulation of metabolite of, 35, 170
    effect on neurotransmission of, 35, 170
    effect on synthesis of norepinephrine, 36,
      170
    general comments on use of, 156, 172
    physiological consequence of accumulation
      of metabolite of, 37
    preparation and mode of administration
      of, 155, 172
    side effects of, 172
  diuretics (thiazide)
    locus and mechanism of action, 177, 180
    dosages, 155
    side effects of, 181
  ganglionic blocking agents, 163-164
    cardiovascular effects, 165
    dosages, 164
    effect on reserpine-induced depletion of
      catecholamine, 166

    use in hypertensive emergencies, 157
  guanethidine
    actions on central nervous system, 176
    adrenergic neuron blocking effect of, 173
    cocaine-like effect of, 173
    depletion of catecholamine stores by, 173
    effect on cardiovascular system, 173
    effect on uptake and retention of norepi-
      nephrine, 17
    general comments on use of, 156, 175
    interaction of drugs with, 176
    preparation and mode of administration
      of, 175
    reserpine-like effect of, 173
    side effects of, 175
  hydralazine
    cardiovascular effects, 182
    general comments on use of, 184
    locus and mechanism of action, 182, 183
    preparations and mode of administration
      of, 182
    toxic effects of, 182
  pargyline
    cardiovascular effects of, 175
    effects on levels of catecholamines, 175
    effects on metabolism of tyramine, 35, 175
    effect on synthesis of norepinephrine, 30
    general comments on use of, 156, 176
    locus and mechanism of action, 35, 175
    preparation and mode of administration
      of, 176
    side effects of, 176
  reserpine
    actions on central nervous system, 164
    antagonism of depleting actions of, 166
    blockade of adrenergic transmission by,
      167
    depletion of catecholamines stores by, 166
    effect on cardiovascular system, 168
    effect on norepinephrine storage particles,
      17
    effect on synthesis of norepinephrine, 167
    effect on retention of norepinephrine, 167
    effect on uptake of norepinephrine, 17-18
    general comments on use of, 169

pharmacological consequences of, 166
preparations and mode of administration of, 169
side effects of, 168-169
time course of recovery after, 167
Axoplasmic transport, 8
colchicine effect on, 9
implication of microtubules in, 9

B

Blood
constituent of, 47
flow of blood, 46
function of, 48
Blood pressure
baroreceptor function in regulation of, 77-83
factors involved in maintenance of, 77-89
hormonal control of, 90, 91
in various parts of the circulation, 59
long term control of, 93
medullary control of, 83-87
sympathetic control of, 83
reflex control of, 80
respiratory control of, 87
role of kidney in regulation of, 93, 94
Blood vessels, 58-76
control of calibre of, 60-73
metabolic, 63
myogenic, 60-62
nervous, 65-73
summary of factors in, 72
innervation of, 65-73
by parasympathetic vasodilator fibers, 18
by sympathetic vasoconstrictor fibers, 65-68
by sympathetic vasodilator fibers, 68
mechanism of vasodilation of, 69
structure
arteries, 58
capillaries, 60
vein, 60

C

Cardiovascular system
adrenergic stimulation effect on, 112
alpha-methyl dopa effect on, 165
angiotensin effect on, 99
control of, 50
division of, 49
exercise effect on, 91-92, 116
ganglionic blocking agents effect on, 165
guanethidine effect on, 173
hydralazine effect on, 182
medullary control of, 83-87
prostaglandin effect on, 119-124
reserpine effect on, 168
sympathomimetic amines, effect on
epinephrine, 119, 121

isoproterenol, 120, 122
norepinephrine, 119, 120
phenylephrine, 123, 124
relative potencies of, 118
Catechol-O-methyltransferase
role in metabolism of catecholamines, 12-15
Catecholamines (see also Norepinephrine)
binding non-specific, 7
classification and structure, 3
complex in storage vesicles, 7
definition and distribution, 3, 4
metabolic disposition, 13, 14
synthesis, 26
Circulation in skin, 73-74
Circulation in skeletal muscle, 74-76

D

Difference between disposition of norepinephrine and epinephrine, 15
Dopamine
structure, 3
distribution, 4
function, 4

E

Epinephrine
structure, 3
distribution, 4
effect on cardiovascular system, 121
function, 4
Exercise, 91, 116
cardiac output during, 91
peripheral resistance and blood pressure during, 92
redistribution of blood during, 92
release of catecholamines during, 91
role of sympathetic nervous system in circulatory response to, 115
synthesis of catecholamines during, 93
venous return during, 92

H

Heart
anatomy and function of, 46-47
contractility and factors affecting, 49-52
effect of coronary perfusion on the performance of, 57
influence of sympathetic nervous system on, 54-55
innervation of
parasympathetic, 53
sympathetic, 54
neural and humoral regulation of **function** of, 56
rate, 48
Starling law of, 50
Hypertension, 127-184
ACTH release and, 134

aldosteronism in, 135
  differences between primary and secondary, 137
  primary, 135
    characteristics of, 137
    clinical symptoms in, 138
  secondary, 135-138
cardiovascular alterations in, 142
choice of drugs in, 152
classification of sustained, 130
control of circumstances in, 144-146
definition, 127
diastolic, 130
drug therapy in management of emergencies in, 157
effect on brain, 148
effect on heart, 148
effect on kidney, 149
effect on retina, 147
essential, 131
factors contributing to adverse prognosis, 150
factors influencing onset and development of, 127
labile, 129
laboratory studies for patients with, 149
malignant, 131
neurogenic, 131-132
oral contraceptive and, 138
program of treatment, 146-157
renal ischemia and, 134
renovascular
  definition of, 140
  diagnostic test for, 139
  indication for medical treatment, 141
  indication for surgical treatment, 140
role of sympathetic nervous system in humans, 142
systolic, 129-130
work sheet for study of patients with, 151

M
Medullary cardiovascular centers, 83-86
  cardio-excitatory center, 83-85
  cardio-exhibitory center, 83-85
  effects of alteration in discharge of, 87
  vasomotor center, 83-85
    factors affecting, 81-82

N
Norepinephrine (catecholamine)
  action on cardiovascular system, 119, 121
  fate of
    bound, 14
    circulating, 13
    in vascular tissue, 21
  in hypotension, 162
  in hypertension, 127-184
  release of, 9-11

by alpha-methyl dopa, 169
by guanethidine, 173
by reserpine, 164
by nerve impulse, 9
by tonic impulses, 9
by tyramine-like drug, 178
calcium role in, 10
false transmitter, effect of, 10
mechanism of, 10
storage in adrenergic neuron, 7
structure and distribution, 3, 4
synthesis, 26-33
  pathway, 27
  rate limiting step in, 28
  regulation of
    through end-product inhibition, 29
    through increased enzyme synthesis, 31
  summary, 32
uptake of, 14-25
  at extraneuronal site, 23-25
    characteristics of, 23
    effect of
      adrenergic blocking drug, 23
      cocaine, 24
      metaraminol, 24
      normetanephrine, 24
      physiological significance, 24-25
  at sympathetic neuronal membrane
    effect of
      adrenergic blocking agents, 24
      antidepressant, 19
      cocaine, 17
      guanethidine, 19
      Ouabaine, 19-20
      temperature, 18
    energy requirement, 18
    ionic requirement, 18
    importance of, 20
    site of binding, 14
    step in, 16
urinary excretion, 13

P
Pheochromocytoma, 158-162
  diagnosis of, 159, 161
  origin of, 158, 159
  pharmacological test, 161
  symptoms of, 159, 160
  treatment of, 161-162
Phenoxybenzamine
  in treatment of pheochromocytoma, 162
  as premedication in surgical removal of pheochromocytoma, 162
Phentolamine
  in treatment of pheochromocytoma, 162
Properties of norepinephrine transport, 18
Prostaglandins, 104-107
  action on heart, 104

action on vascular smooth muscle, 105
distribution, 104
role in hypertension, 106
sympathetic nervous system and, 105

R

Relative importance of binding and metabolism of norepinephrine, 15
Relative importance of catechol-O-methyltransferase and monoamine-oxidase in metabolism of norepinephrine, 13
Renin, 98-103
    function, 103
    regulation of release, 102
    secretion and angiotensin, 101
    secretion and diurnal variation, 103
    secretion and macula densa hypothesis, 101
    secretion and sympathetic nervous system, 101
Role of autonomic nervous system in fainting in response to strong emotions, 87, 88

S

Summary of events at adrenergic neuroeffector organs, 38-42
Sympathetic neuron
    division of, 5, 6
    varicosities in, 6
    storage of norepinephrine in, 7
        mechanisms involved in, 7
Synapse, 5

T

Transmitter
    concept, development of, 4
    false, 34-37
        in hypertension, 176-178
        physiological consequence of accumulation of, 37
        release of norepinephrine, effect of, 36
        synthesis of, 34, 35
        synthesis of norepinephrine, effect of, 36
        uptake of norepinephrine, effect of, 37
Tyrosine hydroxylase
    role in norepinephrine regulation, 28-32